BEAUTY

The New

HAIR

No-rules

STYLE

Beauty Bible

BEAUTY

The New

HAIR

No-rules

STYLE

Beauty Bible

SOPHIE HANNAH

Thorsons

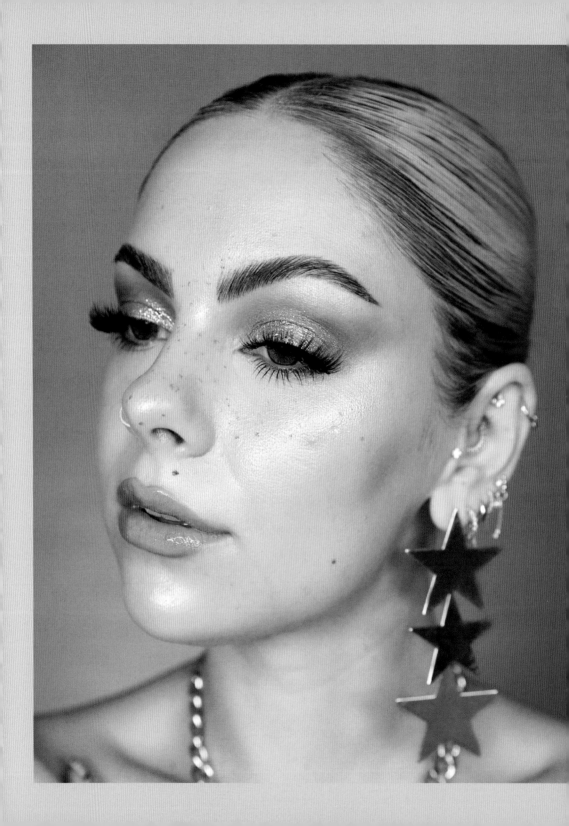

Contents

Introduction

Creative, experimental and self-expressive is how I would describe my style in three words, and I've always been this way. From a young age I was drawn to colour; it started with my bedroom as a child. My mum allowed me to pick the paint and theme and, of course, I chose lilac, neon green and hot pink with swirls, hearts and flowers all over the walls. It was pretty epic! Those were my Tammy Girl days, when I started to pick out my outfits and dress myself, and it was pretty cool to have a mum who allowed me to be myself and dress however I wanted to. That's something that has stayed with me throughout my life; my mum has always supported the way I choose to express myself.

As I got older I was welcomed into the world of makeup at an all-girls' school; and as I've grown up my passion for styling, hair and makeup has evolved. The more I've experimented, the more I've developed my skills in makeup and hair – I've never had one ounce of professional training. My knowledge comes from years of experimenting with different looks in my bedroom at home, taking inspiration from MUAs, watching other content creators on social media and luckily having a sister who's trained in makeup and is on hand to offer tips and tricks.

I'm just your average girl who found a passion for something, but things elevated when I reached an age where I was able to dye my own hair. That was the turning point in my personal style.

Not many people know this, but my career goal was never to become a content creator. It was to become a fashion stylist. I started pursuing this after graduating from university with a fashion photography degree, but I soon found the freelance world to be tough, which then led me to get a job in social media. I worked in London in the industry for a few years and that's when I started my career as a content creator. It didn't happen overnight; I spent those London years setting up a blog and an Instagram account documenting my outfit of the day. It was when my followers kept asking questions about my hair and makeup that I became encouraged to start sharing more of my overall styling looks online, which led me to introduce video tutorials. Fast-forward to today and I can't quite believe I've written a book for you all about beauty, hair and style.

THE CONFIDENCE TO BE *YOU*

This book covers everything from your beauty kit to mastering basic looks and experimenting with colour, right down to dressing for festivals. I'm sharing my experience and knowledge and I really hope by the end of this you have the confidence to be you, to wear makeup for you and to dress for you.

There are no rules when it comes to beauty and fashion – and that's what I love most about it. To me it's an art form, a way you can self-express, share your personality and showcase your creativity. We were all born unique and I think that's an inspiring point to remember when you're next doing your makeup or getting dressed and you're looking at yourself in the mirror. There is nobody out there quite like you. Embrace that!

Remember, life is short. I've learned that from my dad passing away at a young age. If you feel incredible in that dress, wear it! Don't focus on what people 'might' be thinking about you. Although I guarantee that they'd be agreeing with you – that you look incredible.

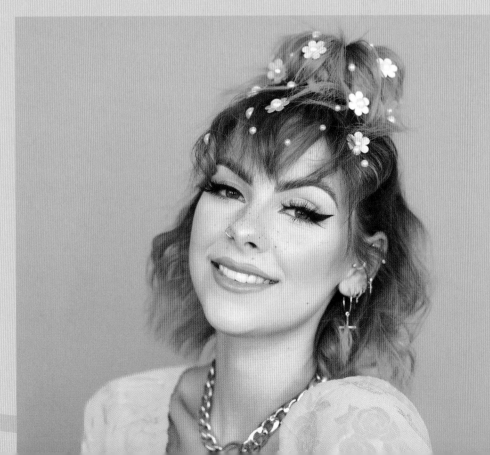

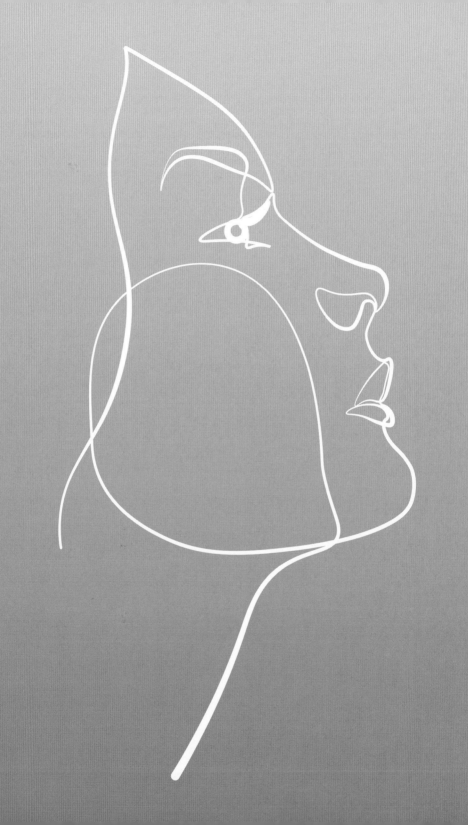

beauty

Let's start with makeup, as it's my first step in getting ready every day.

Makeup Kit

When it comes to makeup your kit is super-important. Using the correct brush for the product you're applying can completely change your look. This is something I've certainly learned through years of doing my own makeup. I never used to even consider what brush I was using to apply products; I would just pick any one from my kit without giving it a second thought. That was until I was chatting to my sister – who is a trained makeup artist – and we got on to the subject of brushes. She showed me her kit and spoke about what she would use each different brush for. The next time I was back in my studio shooting a makeup look, I carefully considered which brush I was picking out. I couldn't believe how much better my makeup looked, all because I was using the right brushes. So, I'm passing what my sister taught me on to you all and I hope it will help you, too.

BRUSHES

Let's talk brushes then. It can be quite overwhelming when you buy a set of brushes, especially when they aren't individually labelled – labelling makes it a whole lot easier. Makeup brushes will help you to create the looks you want; they give you control, help the product application and make it easy when it comes to blending.

I'm going to take you through a complete list of different makeup brushes and their uses. There are so many on the market, but this list will allow you to achieve anything from everyday makeup right through to more creative looks.

FOUNDATION BRUSH

Great for achieving a flawless base with liquid foundations. I personally love the flat style of a foundation brush as it helps me apply the product evenly to my skin, gives me the most control and a full coverage. However, you can find lots of variations; if you like a natural finish to your base makeup, a dense, round-bristle foundation brush might be better for you as it gives a more sheer finish, or use fingers or a beauty blender. It's really down to personal preference and how much coverage you want. My go-to is applying foundation with a brush and finishing off with a beauty blender to soak up any excess and press the product into my skin.

CONCEALER BRUSH

Basically a smaller-scale version of a foundation brush that fits perfectly under the eye. This is a great brush to help you target any areas you want to conceal or highlight. I tend to opt for a beauty blender when applying concealer as I prefer the seamless finish, so you don't get any streaks or lines. A concealer brush is great if you want to build up the coverage, though. You gently pat the product onto your target area, then blend out the edges.

STIPPLING BRUSH

This is great for applying liquid products. It can be used for foundation, tinted moisturiser and cream blush and bronzer. I always opt for a stippling brush for cream bronzer, as it blends product beautifully into the skin and leaves no harsh lines. Because of its design you get a softer airbrushed finish, and it's great for achieving a natural contour.

POWDER BRUSH

These are fluffy and light and tend to vary in size from small to large. I'd recommend having one small and one large in your kit – the small one for setting your undereye and the large for your T-zone. Use with a setting powder and you can load up the product onto the small brush to set your undereye, then add a light dusting over your T-zone with the large brush.

POWDER BRONZER OR BLUSH BRUSH

Now you could have separate brushes for these products, but you really don't need to. As long as the brush is a dome shape with long, fluffy bristles you will be able to seamlessly apply your bronzer and blush. Apply lightly, as this will help you build up the intensity.

CONTOUR BRUSH

Contouring is all about adding dimension to your face. You apply contour product beneath your cheekbones, jawline and on the top of your forehead, and an angled brush will help you with this. If you prefer a sharper look, opt for a brush with blunt bristles, and if you prefer a more natural contour look, find a soft brush.

HIGHLIGHTER BRUSH

Highlighter is one of my favourite things to apply, purely because I love a sparkle and glow. There are quite a few different brushes you could use here: a fan brush, a short dense bristle brush or a long soft bristle brush. I personally prefer a short dense bristle brush as I find it helps me build my highlighter and really buff it into my base.

BROW BRUSH

This is a small, dense, firm and angled brush. This can be used to define and fill in your brows and even create hair-like strokes using a brow pomade. I'd highly recommend getting a double-ended brow brush that has a spoolie on the end, as this is great for brushing brows through before applying product, or for helping push your brow hairs into place after using a brow gel.

FLAT EYESHADOW BRUSH

A dense, rounded-tip brush that's really going to pack on your eyeshadow. This will help you to build the intensity of your eyeshadow colour on your lid. You can also use this to apply eyeshadow under your bottom lash line.

EYESHADOW BLENDING BRUSH

This is going to help you get an amazing, flawless blend of your eyeshadow. Use a blending brush after you have packed on your eyeshadow colour to blend out the edges and crease or, if you've used multiple colours, to blend them into one another. Use this brush bare, with no product on, to achieve a seamless blend. When it comes to blending eyeshadow, I also like to have a small eyeshadow blending brush to hand. This helps buff the very edge of your eyeshadow blend and also any shadow you've applied under your bottom lash line.

EYESHADOW CREASE BRUSH

Another favourite brush, and if you get this brush right your cut creases are going to be on point. This brush is flat, very dense and sharply rounded. It needs to be sharp so when you're cutting your crease it's precise. I also use this style of brush to carve the underneath of my brows to make them sharper.

EYELINER BRUSH

Even if you opt for a liquid liner product over applying a gel liner with a brush you should definitely have an eyeliner brush in your kit. It will come in handy if you ever fancy getting creative. I use a thin, sharp brush for all my intricate eye looks – it really helps with fine line detailing. If you do love to apply eyeliner with a brush, a small, sharp-angled brush can help you achieve a precise wing and lash line. You could also double up your brow brush as an eyeliner brush.

LIP BRUSH

I love a lip brush; it gives me more precision when applying a liquid lip, and on occasions I can get away without needing a lip liner. I also use this brush when I'm blending out a lighter lip colour in the centre of my lips. A lip brush tends to be a smaller version of what a concealer brush looks like; it's got a sharp edge for defining your cupid's bow and lip shape but the brush is soft so you can blend your lip liner shade seamlessly into your lip colour.

I've tried a lot of brushes on the market, but my recommendations for a good place to start your brush kit are:

Zoeva
Mykitco.
Spectrum
e.l.f. Cosmetics
Real Techniques
Eco Tools

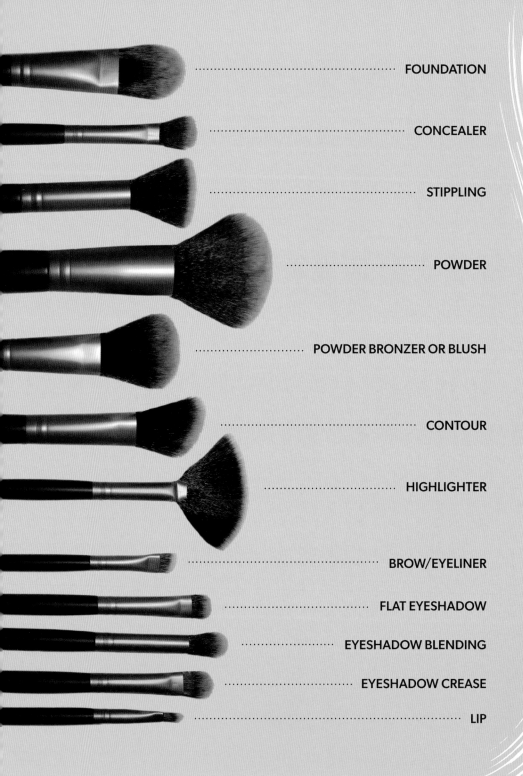

FOUNDATION

CONCEALER

STIPPLING

POWDER

POWDER BRONZER OR BLUSH

CONTOUR

HIGHLIGHTER

BROW/EYELINER

FLAT EYESHADOW

EYESHADOW BLENDING

EYESHADOW CREASE

LIP

Now you've got your brushes sorted, there are a few more things in your kit that you will find super-useful – some that you will be using every day and some for when you might be doing something more creative with your makeup. Don't feel you need to run to the shop as soon as you've read through this list – a kit is something you build up over time. What might be useful to me might be useless to you, so think about what your key items are to kick-start your makeup kit, then add to it whenever you want to.

MAKEUP SPONGES

This is a great example of where your kit might differ to other people's. When it comes to applying foundation I start with a foundation brush, but I like to finish with a makeup sponge to really work it into the skin and remove any excess product. Some might prefer using fingers or just a brush for their foundation application. Same with concealer; everyone will have a way that works for them when it comes to applying and working it into the skin. It's definitely personal preference and will take some experimenting, but that's what I love about makeup, it's about you and what makes you feel good. You don't need to apply your makeup the same way as everyone else.

SCISSORS

This might be pretty obvious, but definitely invest in a pair of mini lash and brow scissors. If you wear false lashes like me, they tend to be longer than my lash line and I always have to trim them. With brows, you can keep these shaped at home as lash and brow scissors have a slight curved blade that will follow your natural arch.

TWEEZERS

Following on from scissors, a great pair of sharp tweezers is always handy if you're wanting to get rid of any stray hairs or define your brows. I actually like to use tweezers to apply my false lashes, or if I'm wearing mascara and a few lashes have clumped together, tweezers work wonders at separating them.

EYELASH APPLICATOR

If you're nervous about putting tweezers near your eyes, which I feel like I should be, you can invest in an eyelash applicator. This is designed like a pair of tweezers but the end has a curved tip that gently and securely holds the false lashes. Once you've applied your glue, you can fix them straight onto your lash line.

EYELASH CURLERS

Still on lashes! If you prefer wearing mascara over false eyelashes, I would highly recommend an eyelash curler tool. It's super-easy to use and it gives your lashes a lift before applying mascara. It's a game changer!

LASH COMB

One final lash tool you might find useful is a lash comb. Again, if you're a mascara wearer a lash comb will separate your lashes and add volume. However, you should be able to find a good mascara on the market that does this for you.

SHARPENER

A product I always misplace in my kit (but that is so needed) is a sharpener for your lip and eye pencils. I recommend having a universal one that has two different-sized pencil holes and comes with a removable case to hold the shavings. I love that feeling when you're using a blunt lip liner and think 'oh this needs sharpening'. You sharpen it, use it and, wow, it really makes a difference!

FACE RAZOR

This is specifically designed for use on your face – it kind of looks like a scalpel but it's super-gentle on your skin. It minimises the appearance of all that peach fuzz and can also exfoliate to remove dead skin cells in a process known as dermaplaning, which in turn can brighten your skin and help your makeup apply more smoothly and last longer. It's a tool not everyone will choose to use, because facial hair is absolutely normal and not an issue, but I love a face razor. I use it on my cheeks, for shaping my brows and hairline and removing unwanted hair from my upper lip. I personally love the way my foundation sits on my face after I defuzz my skin.

EMBELLISHMENT APPLICATOR

I do a lot of creative looks and one thing I get asked all the time is how I apply embellishment. I use an applicator that's double-ended – one end has a pointed wax tip and the other is stainless steel to make sure the embellishment – such as rhinestones – are secure and in position. This tool is universal, as it's also used for nail art.

MIXING PALETTE

The final item I'd recommend having in your kit is a makeup mixing palette. It's so useful if you're mixing foundation shades to complement your complexion, or if you love experimenting with colour combinations.

I've probably overwhelmed you with this list, but as I said, a kit is something you build up over time. It's an investment. Some brushes or tools can be quite costly and they do add up, so I'd definitely recommend starting with a few must-have items, then over time you can decide which of the other items you need.

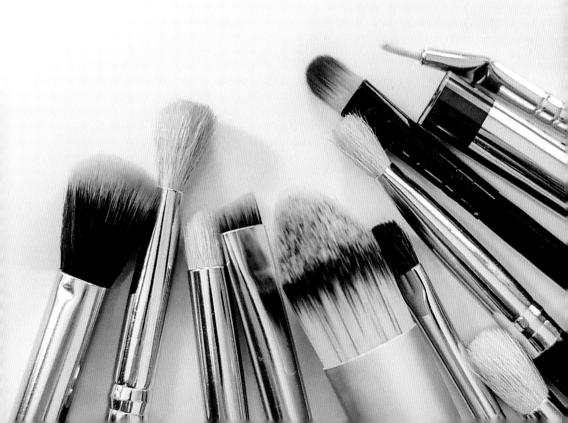

CLEANING YOUR KIT

So once you've built your kit and started using all your tools, there will come a day where you need to clean everything. I think we're all guilty of leaving our makeup brushes for weeks without cleaning, but they collect so much bacteria from your skin, in the air and where you store them, and using them while dirty can lead to breakouts.

There is nothing better than freshly cleaned makeup brushes and sponges, and it actually helps with your makeup application as well. For example, your foundation brush can become somewhat stiff if it hasn't been cleaned and you won't get such a smooth finish. I've tried and tested a few ways of cleaning my kit and I'm going to share my top tips with you.

There are tons of products on the market for cleaning brushes, from bars that are essentially like soap to liquid cleaners. I used to stand over my bathroom sink for hours using a cleaning bar and washing my brushes one by one. It's a rather tedious task, then you are brushless for a day or so while you wait for them to fully dry. However, this job got a lot easier when I discovered an incredible product from Cinema Secrets. It's a professional brush cleaner that can be used on natural and synthetic brushes, it removes 99.9% of bacteria and you don't need to rinse it off! It's a game changer. I pour a little into a small container, enough to cover about a quarter of the bristles on a brush, dip the brush in, then wipe it on a clean cloth or paper towel. You will see your brush clean within seconds in front of your eyes – and the best part, it's also DRY! So if you're doing a makeup look where you need to use multiple eyeshadow colours you can have your brushes clean and dry in between each colour within seconds. It's great if you're being sustainable with your kit as you won't need to buy five of the same eye brush.

When it comes to cleaning your makeup sponges there are a few ways to do this – it kind of comes down to what's most convenient for you. One easy way is with soap and warm water, which you can do over your bathroom sink. First hold your sponge under warm running water, then massage the soap into the sponge, working it in with your fingers and making sure it all soaks in. Rinse, and while rinsing gently squeeze the sponge to make sure all the leftover makeup and dirt is out. When it comes to picking a soap there are a lot out there on the market, including speciality liquid or bar ones, but washing-up liquid also works a treat and is less expensive.

If your sponge is on the dirtier side and you can't remember when you last cleaned it, it might need a little more work – and giving it a soak in warm water and soap might be the better option. Liquid soap works best for this. Soak the sponge in a small tub or bowl for a few minutes, then squeeze it a few times. Add some more soap, massage, then rinse under running warm water.

The method I find is the most thorough and the most convenient is chucking my sponges in with my clothes wash. You will need a little net bag for this, which you'll already have if you use reusable makeup pads. It's super-easy to do, although it takes a little longer as a wash tends to be on for a few hours, but when it's done my sponge is like new.

Your makeup brushes and sponges aren't the only things in your kit that need maintenance, there are other tools that get a build-up of makeup and bacteria that should be cleaned after use. For example, eyelash curlers get a coating of mascara, and if they're not cleaned, they actually become harder to use. They also need to be clean because they get used really close to your lash line, which is a delicate area prone to styes and infections. Having biodegradable makeup wipes or reusable makeup pads and makeup remover on hand is really useful, so either straight after you've used a tool or before you use it you can give it a quick wipe. Having a little spray bottle of 70% alcohol on your dressing table is another great idea, to just give your tools a quick spritz so they are getting a further disinfect after you've cleaned them.

Cleaning your kit might not be the most exciting thing in the world but it's important to protect your skin and eyes from bacteria, and once you've done it, it really does feel nice to sit down with sparkly clean brushes ready for another makeup look.

'Makeup kit cleaning and organising is a neverending story. I change over my kit depending on the job – what I take for fashion week is very different to what I take for TV or bridal, for example. Normally before a big event like fashion week I take out my entire kit; refill travel-size bottles, sanitise products with 70% isopropyl alcohol and check everything is labelled correctly. My personal makeup bag is a little less organised but I like to keep it clean so when I deep clean my kit I also give my personal products a wipe over! Brushes for clients are washed after every use, it's part of my evening ritual to give them a bath. Having clean tools (brushes, sponges, etc.) can also really impact your base makeup application, as if you haven't washed your personal brush in weeks it's going to be filled with oils that can break down your makeup.'

HANNAH BENNETT, MAC SENIOR ARTIST

STORING YOUR KIT

I don't know about you, but I find storing and organising all of my beauty products and tools so satisfying. Separating everything into categories, getting my label-maker out and decorating my dressing table – it can be so rewarding when everything is organised. It makes it so much easier while doing your makeup if you know where everything is and it's easily accessible.

There are so many options when it comes to storing your makeup kit. You might have a dressing table with a number of drawers so you could use draw dividers, or you might prefer having all of your kit on display in a storage box or desk organiser. My kit is vast, so I tend to use both options. I have numerous drawers that I have divided into makeup categories such as foundation and concealer, powders, eyeliner, mascara, and so on. Each category gets its own labelled drawer, within which dividers then keep everything separate and organised. I can get carried away with a label-maker!

When it comes to storing makeup brushes, I like to have these out in front of me and visible so I can quickly grab the right brush for the right application. There are so many options for storing makeup brushes – you might buy a set of brushes that come with a storage box or roll-up case – in which case if you wanted to be sustainable you wouldn't need to invest in a brush holder.

The majority of dressing-table organisers and brush holders are made of acrylic, and although that's not very eco-friendly, they have longevity because it's a durable material and really easy to keep clean.

However, you might be a DIY queen or interiors junkie and want to think outside of the box about other ways you could store your beauty products, especially in a more sustainable way. I've seen numerous upcycling ideas online like using small plant pots, repurposing baked bean cans or even using burnt-out glass candles for storing brushes.

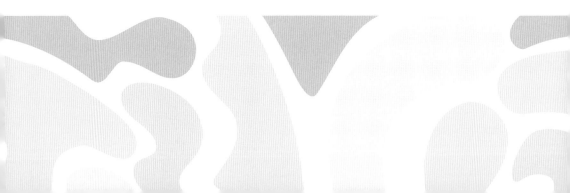

Mastering Your Everyday Base Makeup

Base makeup is such a personal preference, and with there being a vast amount of products on the market, it can be quite overwhelming. You need to do your base makeup the way you like it – whether that's not wearing it or wanting to achieve a flawless, full-coverage look.

Everyone's skin is unique, and how one person creates their base might not be right for your skin. The base is the core of your makeup looks – think of it like building a house: you have your prep (skincare), the foundations (your base makeup), the structure (contour/blush/highlight/brows) and the decorating (eyes/lips). You need your foundations to be strong for the rest of your makeup to sit right.

I'm going to take you through how you can master your everyday base makeup. It might take some trial and error – I know I tried numerous foundations and concealers before finding the one I'm happy with – but hopefully this guide will give you a good starting point that you can take away and work on as you become more confident.

THE PREP – SKINCARE

If you want to ensure your makeup stays on throughout the day and looks just as good in the evening as when you left the house that morning, you need to prep your skin first. If you skip the prep you could end up with dry patches or uneven coverage by the end of the day, and who wants that when they've spent time perfecting that blend?

'You can spend a fortune on expensive makeup products that are long-wear or full-coverage with all of these amazing things, but if you do not look after your skin nothing is going to sit on your skin properly. If you want to get the most out of your makeup products you need to start with your skin.'

KATIE BRANCH,
MUA MAKEUP ACADEMY

1. CLEANSE

Before you start prepping your skin you want to make sure your skin is clean. Using a gentle cleanser – a favourite of mine is the Elemis Cleansing Balm – gently massage it into your skin to remove any dirt, oil and impurities, then rinse with lukewarm water. If you've cleansed the night before, you don't necessarily need to do this step, you can just splash your face with warm water. It'll depend on your skin type and whether you want to clean off all the moisturisers or serums you used in your nighttime routine.

2. EXFOLIATE

This step should be done 2–3 times a week. Exfoliating your face cleans and purifies clogged pores, evens skin tone, helps skincare products penetrate deeper and boosts circulation. Ideally, do this step straight after cleansing; so once you have rinsed off your cleanser, gently massage an exfoliator product into your skin in a circular motion. Then rinse again with lukewarm water. Your skin should feel silky and smooth at this point. I have a few favourite exfoliating products but my top two have to be the Ole Henriksen Lemonade Smoothing Scrub and the Huda Beauty Yo Enzyme Scrub. Both leave my skin soft and flawless and I see a huge difference immediately.

3. TONER

Toning comes after cleansing, unless it's your exfoliating day. A toner will help get rid of any leftover impurities and will leave your skin feeling refreshed and ready for your main skincare products: serum, eye cream and moisturiser. Take a toner of your choice and apply to a clean reusable makeup pad, then gently blot all over the face. Toners can be used once or twice a day, depending on how often you cleanse.

4. SERUM

I love a serum, and now that you've done the first three steps a serum will really penetrate deep into your skin. What your skin needs will be judged by you, so if you feel your skin is dehydrated you want a serum containing hyaluronic acid. If you're after anti-ageing, look for retinol in the formula, and if you're after smoothing and brightening, find a serum with vitamin C. A serum is where you can target your skincare concerns, so really look into the ingredients to pick the right one for you and your skin type.

5. EYE CREAM

Eye creams are specially formulated for your eye area, where the skin is completely different to the rest of your face: it is much thinner and more delicate and is the first area to show dryness. This means it's easier to see discoloration here. As with your serum, you need to choose an eye cream that's right for you and your skin concerns. You might want to target fine lines and wrinkles, for which ingredients such as retinol, vitamin C and hyaluronic acid are great, or if you have puffiness, caffeine as an ingredient works wonders.

Make sure you apply your chosen eye cream before your moisturiser and gently pat the product under and around your eye up to your brow bone. Using your ring finger works well for the application of an eye cream (make sure your hands are clean).

6. MOISTURISE

Probably my favourite part of my skincare prep before applying my makeup. You will need to find a moisturiser that works well for your skin type and keeps your skin hydrated and refreshed throughout the day. A moisturiser essentially acts as a barrier between your skin and the weather that could dry it out. A top tip is don't rub moisturiser into your skin, press it in, as it will seep into your skin better that way. When choosing a moisturiser, if your skin is dry opt for a cream, and if your skin is oily opt for a lightweight cream or gel. The handy thing about finding a moisturiser for your skin concern is most of them will reference it on the packaging – so if you're more on the oily side, look for oil-free products.

7. SPF!

Never miss out this step, it's so important to take care of your skin and protect it against harsh sun while you're out and about, regardless of the season. The sun's UV rays are still strong in winter, and even if you can't see the sun it can still do damage to your skin if you're not looking after it. Wait for your moisturiser to penetrate before applying your SPF and be sure to top up throughout the day using an SPF mist that can go over makeup.

The choice of SPFs can be quite overwhelming. You will want to choose one specifically for the face and that targets any skin concerns or sensitivity. I also recommend opting for factor 50+, as this is going to give your skin the highest protection. A few favourite brands of mine for SPF are Garnier and Ultra Violette.

8. PRIMER

Once these important skincare steps are complete, you're not going to want to miss applying a primer. A primer helps to create a smooth canvas and ensures your makeup will last throughout the day. Always think about what your desired finished look is before applying a primer. Do you want a matte finish or a glowy look? There are so many options out there, so again you should find one that works with your skin concerns. For example, if you find your skin gets dry opt for a hydrating primer, or if your skin is oily opt for a mattifying primer to help with shininess. I tend to use a colour-correcting primer to combat any redness and uneven skin tone. Smashbox's range of Photo Finish primers are great, in particular Reduce Redness – it's been formulated with ingredients to protect your skin and the green tone does exactly as its name suggests.

9. LIPS

Don't forget about your lips, they're part of your skin too. I suffer with dry lips and on the days when I skip this step I always find my lipstick cracks and flakes. Once a week I exfoliate my lips and every day I apply a lip primer. Lip primers help hydrate and up the longevity and staying power of your chosen lip colour.

'Growing up, makeup to me was seen as a mask, so I sadly didn't enjoy it. But the only reason I saw it as a mask is because I had cystic acne and felt like I had to cover my skin to function. I wouldn't leave the house without makeup, I wouldn't even go downstairs to see my parents without makeup. Because of the images of "perfect" skin in the media I felt like I to needed to look like that, however I was so wrong! It wasn't until I created #freethepimple and really just let myself free my skin did I find out that the "perfect" image in the media isn't real and DOESN'T exist. I realised that I can go makeup-free even with acne, and makeup is there for me to enjoy and, yes, it can help cover things up and give you confidence but don't let it take over, and don't let it be a mask. Have fun with makeup and remember it's not going to make you poreless and flawless, because that doesn't exist, lovelies!'
LOU NORTHCOTE, CONTENT CREATOR

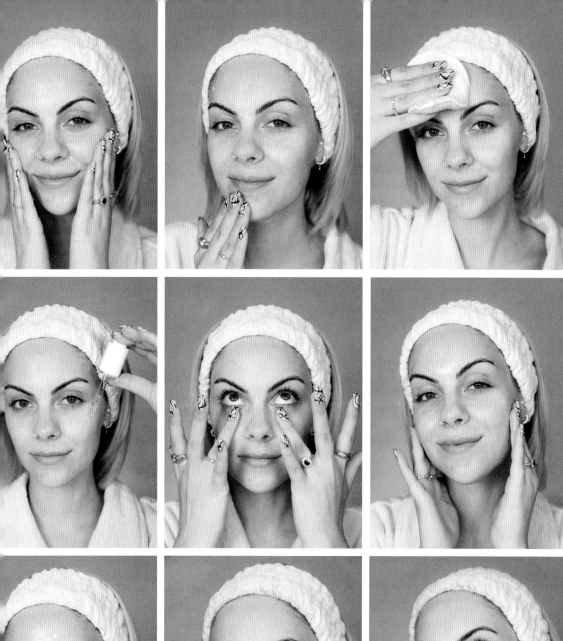
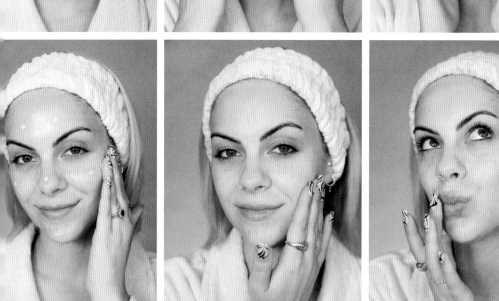

FOUNDATION AND CONCEALER

After you've completed your skincare routine, you're ready to jump in and create your base makeup. I want to start by saying none of us 'need' base makeup, our skin is real and beautiful and we don't have to hide pigmentation or a skin condition. There's also no shame in wanting to cover or enhance our natural skin for certain looks either – you do whatever makes you feel good and confident.

Choosing a foundation and concealer depends on your skin concerns, how you want your skin to look, your skin type, tone and colour. There are a lot of factors to consider, so I hope my guide below can help you to pick the right products for you.

Getting the right makeup is important to prevent breakouts and irritation, and your face ending up a different tone to the rest of your skin. I think we've all been there. I've definitely had times in my teenage years where I experimented with makeup and ended up with orange circles under my eyes from trying to conceal my undereye redness but chose the wrong shade of concealer. Or my face has been a totally different colour to my neck and I've got a foundation line from not blending under my jawline. Makeup is something you get better at over the years through experimenting and figuring out what works for you.

Let's start with foundation:

CHOOSING YOUR COVERAGE AND FINISH

The first consideration when it comes to picking your foundation and concealer is 'coverage' – what areas of concern you have and how much of your natural skin you want to show or cover. Products will state what level of coverage they are for. Here's a rundown of what they mean:

My top picks:

Light/sheer coverage, glowy finish:
e.l.f. Halo Glow Liquid Filter

Medium coverage:
Shiseido Synchro Skin Self-refreshing Foundation

Full coverage, matte finish:
Charlotte Tilbury Airbrush Flawless Foundation

MAKEUP-FREE – you might not be a foundation or concealer wearer, so once you've done your skincare routine and added SPF, you can go straight ahead and apply the makeup you love to wear, if any! Just don't forget to prime if you're adding any sculpting, highlighter or blush.

LIGHT/SHEER COVERAGE – this is for those who want to enhance their natural skin. Maybe you have freckles you don't want to conceal? Within this category you don't only have foundation to choose from, you also have BB and CC creams (see below), skin tints and tinted moisturisers.

MEDIUM COVERAGE – for those who want to even out skin tone and prefer a formula that's buildable to achieve the coverage they desire without it feeling too heavy on the skin. This tends to be the coverage I opt for with my everyday base makeup.

FULL COVERAGE – this is for you if you want to completely even out your skin tone and fully hide areas of concern like blemishes. Full coverage might be something you opt for every day or just on select occasions, such as if you are going to a special event or a photo shoot, because some people might find full coverage can cause clogged pores. I use full coverage from time to time, especially for any glam looks. When it comes to concealer, I always opt for a full coverage to conceal my undereye redness.

You will also want to consider the finish you want. A natural finish gives a light effect so your skin still looks like your skin; a matte finish is shine-free and is a good option if your skin is oily; while a dewy finish creates glowy, radiant skin, which is a popular choice if you have dry skin.

'When applying foundation, I like to work in thin layers to build up coverage rather than applying one thick coat to the skin. Using colour correctors also allows you to hide any areas like dark circles, redness or pigmentation without using lots of coverage. The skin is multidimensional and doesn't contain only one tone or shade, so when we use just one foundation it can look dull and flat – but of course most people don't want to buy multiple shades of foundation, so that's where contour highlight and blush come in handy!'

**HANNAH BENNETT,
MAC SENIOR ARTIST**

TYPES OF FOUNDATIONS

Moving on to types of foundations, these come in a variety of different formulas, each offering different benefits, coverage and finishes. With so many on the market, you will be able to find one that's specific to you.

LIQUID FOUNDATION – the most popular foundation, this comes in a wide range of formulas and consistencies, offering anything from light to fuller coverage, alongside different finishes from glowy to matte.

MOUSSE FOUNDATION – this formulation contains air so it is super-lightweight on the skin and can offer a full coverage.

FOUNDATION STICK – offers full coverage and is mess-free. You're not going to have a foundation explosion in your handbag with this.

MINERAL FOUNDATION – contains minerals from the earth and is free from preservatives, fragrance and dyes, meaning it's kinder to sensitive skin.

POWDER FOUNDATION – comes in a compact case so it's super-convenient and super-buildable. You can wear this alone or over the top of a liquid foundation for a fuller coverage.

BB CREAM – 'BB' stands for beauty balm or blemish balm. Great for that 'no-makeup' makeup look. It has added ingredients that you often find in skincare, so you can cover blemishes but also care for your skin.

CC CREAM (COLOUR CONTROL OR COMPLEXION CORRECTOR) – is a slightly lighter formula that has everything a BB cream has but focuses more on anti-ageing properties, with ingredients such as vitamin B3 (niacinamide) as this reduces the look of wrinkles and improves the skin's surface.

TINTED MOISTURISER – has a sheer, light coverage and is great for achieving a dewy complexion.

WHAT WORKS FOR YOUR SKIN TYPE?

Oily skin – try a matte powder foundation, oil-free liquid foundation and CC cream.

Dry skin – moisturising liquid, cream and mousse foundations or a BB cream are great. Opt for a dewy finish to avoid any dry patches.

Combination skin – liquid or powder foundation both work well.

Mature skin – water-based liquid foundations are great; avoid powder or stick foundations as these will highlight wrinkles and fine lines.

Skin conditions:

Eczema – formulas free from triggers like parabens, fragrances, preservatives, and propylene glycol. Look for lightweight foundations with ingredients such as hyaluronic acid and glycerin.

Psoriasis – steer clear of matte finishes and opt for formulas that are creamy and hydrating.

Rosacea – opt for foundations that have anti-inflammatory and anti-redness ingredients.

Cystic acne – hydrating foundations work great especially if they're packed with antioxidant ingredients like vitamin C, which can help to leave skin brighter and to fade acne scarring. A CC cream also works well for acne.

CHOOSING A CONCEALER THAT'S RIGHT FOR YOU

Choosing a concealer also depends on what facial feature you want to target and your skin type. Maybe you want to cover acne, dark spots, pigmentation or the undereye area? Concealer will do the job and a little will go a long way.

There are many types of concealer to choose from:

LIQUID CONCEALER – the most versatile option, a liquid product provides the best hydration and gives medium to full coverage. Great for acne-prone skin, because it allows your skin to breathe.

PENCIL CONCEALER – makes it super-easy to cover an unsightly spot. This type of concealer gives a light to full coverage and it's easy to carry around with you and touch up on the go.

PEN CONCEALERS – a liquid concealer in the form of a pen applicator with a button that you press to release the concealer onto the brush. It's practical and great for concealing and brightening the undereye area. These tend to provide light to full coverage.

CREAM CONCEALER – highly pigmented and provides a full coverage. Great for covering blemishes and scars.

COLOUR-CORRECTING CONCEALER – this goes under foundation and helps by counteracting discoloured undertones on your skin. Knowing what colour to use is the key here:

Green concealer – for redness, acne and rosacea
Orange concealer – for darker skin tones
Pink concealer – for fair skin tones with dark circles
Yellow concealer – dark-purple bruises, veins and undereye area
Purple concealer – for yellow skin tones to brighten skin

STICK CONCEALER – medium to full coverage, great for the undereye area and super-easy to apply and blend.

CREAM TO POWDER CONCEALER – you apply this as a cream and it sets as a powder. Great for those with oily skin.

My top picks:
Affordable: NYX Cosmetics HD Photogenic Concealer Wand
Mid-range: HNB Cosmetics Soft Focus Airbrush Concealer
High-end: Shiseido Synchro Skin Self-refreshing Concealer
Sustainable: ZAO Vegan Liquid Concealer

USING A CONCEALER

To get the most out of your concealer, it's all about placement. Not only is concealer used for blemishes, discoloration and under eyes, it can also be used to sculpt the face and highlight features. When choosing a concealer, pick one that's one or two shades lighter than your skin tone.

The areas you might want to conceal are:
- Undereye
- Around the nose
- Spots, blemishes or scars
- The centre of the chin

The areas you might want to highlight are:
- The centre of the forehead
- Down the bridge of your nose
- Under your brow on the arch
- On your cheekbones
- Inner eye

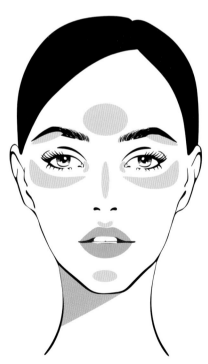

HOW TO FIND THE RIGHT SHADE FOR YOUR SKIN TONE AND COLOUR

Once you know your skin type, tone, undertone and the level of coverage you desire in your foundation/concealer, you can select your product and find the right shade. A lot of brands will have many shades within their ranges – some have a wider selection than others so you can select a shade that works not only with your skin tone but also your undertone.

Your skin tone is the first thing you see – fair, light, medium, dark, deep or somewhere in between. That's pretty simple to figure out, what's a little trickier is working out your undertone, but I've got a handy tip for that. Check your veins on your wrist in natural light, if you have blue or purple veins you have a cool undertone; green veins indicate a warm undertone; while a mix of blue and green veins mean a neutral undertone.

Once you have your skin tone sorted, you can select the right shade for you – I highly recommend sampling a few shades of foundation and blending them onto your cheek to find the perfect match. You will know straight away that it's right if it blends seamlessly into your skin.

If you're still having trouble finding your shade there are so many other ways you can figure it out, either by popping into a local store and getting colour matched with the exact foundation you want or, thanks to great technology, some makeup-brand websites have shade finders where you can digitally upload a photo of your face and it will figure out your shade.

Another site I like to use is findation.com – it's especially good if you already know your shade in one brand but want to switch to another.

APPLYING FOUNDATION AND CONCEALER

Once you've found the perfect shade and formula for your skin, the way your foundation will look will depend on your application. Refer back to the makeup tools section (see page 10) to try out a few ways of applying your base to find what you prefer. I like to use a foundation brush to apply it to my skin as I find you can achieve more coverage this way. But then I like to finish off with a makeup sponge to remove any excess and work the product into the skin.

Mastering foundation and concealer will take some trial and error, but you will get there. There are a lot of factors that can alter over time, however, such as skin changes or brands adjusting their formula, so sometimes you might find your go-to base makeup just isn't working for you anymore. If that's the case, hopefully with my tips above you can easily get back to the perfect base.

BUILDING YOUR BASE

Once you've mastered foundation and concealer, it's time to build on your base – I'm talking contouring, setting, highlight, blusher and brows. Again, how you finish your base will depend on the overall look you're wanting to achieve and even on the occasion. That's one thing I love about makeup, all the different looks you can achieve. I have a go-to way of doing my makeup for everyday but when it comes to festivals, holidays, attending a wedding or maybe just matching my outfit, I switch up how I finish off my base makeup.

Makeup is experimental and there really are no rules, but there are a few tricks and ways you can strategically apply products that will help you to showcase your best features.

'As a makeup artist we learn to contour with cool tones because the contour should look like a natural shadow in the skin, therefore shades of grey and taupe are ideal. It also needs to be matte. When something is shiny it reflects the light and appears more forward to the eye, when it's matte and dark it seems more pushed-back. You can of course use bronzers, but normally I sculpt the face first with a cool tone to create dimension, then add a bronzer on top for warmth if necessary.'
HANNAH BENNETT, MAC SENIOR ARTIST

CONTOURING

This is your next step after you've applied foundation and concealer. Contouring is about adding dimension to your face by sculpting its shape to enhance certain areas. It's about working with a deeper shade to your foundation to add depth or create a stronger jawline or prominent cheekbones.

My top picks:
Affordable: *e.l.f. Cosmetics Putty Bronzer*
Mid-range: *KASH Beauty Bronze Sculpt Stick*
High-end: *Anastasia Beverly Hills Cream Bronzer*
Sustainable: *Lily Lolo Bronzer*

There are two ways to sculpt: using a cream or powder bronzer. If you opt for a powder bronzer you should set your concealer before you do this step. If you use a cream you can do this straight after you've applied your concealer.

There are so many different techniques you can use to contour. The most common is by drawing lines in the areas you want to sculpt using your chosen deeper shade of cream bronzer and then buffing it out. However, I find this technique is good for nose contour but not for the rest of the face as it can sometimes look quite harsh on the skin, and you might also apply too much product.

I find using a cream bronzer and adding the product to your brush before applying it in your chosen areas works best and looks most natural. You can then build up the depth more easily. With the brush you use more of a dabbing application on your facial areas, which will help buff into your foundation and look seamless.

If you prefer a powder bronzer over cream, apply the product to your brush and gently build up the depth by buffing it into the skin. You can use a bronzer brush for facial areas and an angled blending brush works well for the nose.

Contouring can be quite tricky to start with, mainly knowing where to add the depth. You need to figure out what face and nose shape you have, which can be done by looking at yourself in the mirror (see contour guide below). Once you've figured this out you can sculpt your face to really emphasise your features. My guide will help you with this.

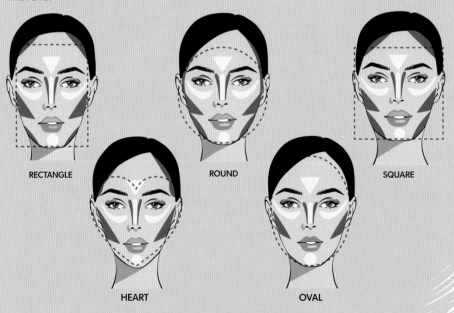

RECTANGLE   ROUND   SQUARE

HEART   OVAL

BLUSH

Following on from sculpting we have blush, which helps to shape your face. Blush can completely change your look; it can add a rosy glow or it can lift your cheekbones. Just as with contouring, you can opt for a liquid/cream blush or a powder. If you opt for a liquid/cream blush you want to apply this before you set your base.

My top picks:
Affordable: XX Revolution XXcess Blush Powder
Mid-range: Benefit Cosmetics Mini Blush
High-end: Dior Backstage Rosy Glow
Sustainable: Lily Lolo Blush

When it comes to choosing a blush colour there are shades to suit everyone's skin tone:

Light/fair skin – soft pinks to peachy corals
Medium skin – rich pinks to cherry
Dark skin – warm pinks/peaches to deep purples

However, these are just guidelines; you might want to experiment and switch things up – for example, if you know you're going to pick a specific eyeshadow colour, you might want to choose a blush to complement it.

When it comes to blush placement, again, this totally depends on your face shape. I wasn't a blush wearer until recently and now I can't leave the house without it. It just gives my face colour and really enhances its shape.

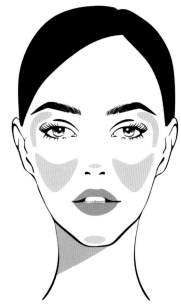

I prefer to opt for a powder blush over a liquid/cream as I find it easier to build up the colour and blend it out using a blusher brush. So I apply blush after setting powder, but if you're opting for a cream/liquid blush, apply this before you set your base.

Here's an easy-to-follow guide for where to place your blush to enhance your face shape.

SETTING

If you've opted for a liquid or cream foundation, concealer, bronzer/blush you're going to want to set your face so these products stay in place all day. This is one of the most important steps in your makeup routine as this is what is going to give your look longevity and a smoother finish. It's also a great step to include if your skin is oily, as you can strategically place setting powder onto your T-zone to absorb excess oil.

With setting powder, less is more. You don't need to load up your brush, it's best to pat your brush into the powder and tap off any excess before you apply it. This way you can build it up to the matte finish you desire. With the application I tend to focus on my undereye, nose, forehead, chin and the sides of the mouth.

When picking a setting powder you can either go for translucent – a white powder that applies invisibly – or one with a coloured tint. Ideally, if you're happy with your foundation/concealer and bronzer application I'd opt for a translucent, as this won't affect your base and will just mattify and lock it in place.

There are a lot of tinted setting powders to pick from, which can help brighten, neutralise or add warmth to your skin tone. Or if you want to achieve an even fuller coverage, pick a setting powder close to your skin tone to keep building on your base.

Once your base is set you can go in and apply your blush if you didn't opt for a cream/liquid formula, and use a powder bronzer to enhance your contouring.

HIGHLIGHTER

Probably my favourite step – I am obsessed with a glow! This is another product that comes in a cream, liquid or powder formula, so pick whichever one works for you depending on the overall finish you desire.

If you want that wet, natural, glowy finish, try an illuminator and apply it with a beauty sponge – your skin will look like glass! An illuminator is a liquid product that gives your skin a natural glow, as opposed to a highlighter, which is more concentrated to your high points. What I love most about an illuminator is how versatile it is; you can mix it in with your moisturiser for no-makeup days to give your skin a radiant glow, or even with your foundation.

I like a glow, but in a powder finish, so I always choose a powder highlighter. I love that there are so many different shades of highlighter on the market. You can go for a more golden glow or find ones that have an iridescent hue. I switch up my highlighter depending on what look I'm doing; if I'm on holiday I love that golden sunkissed look, but if I'm at a festival I love to match my highlight to my outfit, which could be purple, pink or blue.

My top picks:
Affordable: *e.l.f. cosmetics Baked Highlighter*
Mid-range: *Sleek MakeUP Cleopatra's Kiss Highlighting Palette*
High-end: *Benefit Cookie Powder Highlighter*
Sustainable: *ZAO Shine-Up Powder*

When it comes to applying highlighter, stick to the parts of your face that catch the light – you essentially want to highlight your natural high-point features. A top tip on where to place your highlighter is to grab a mirror, get in front of a window in natural light, be bare-faced and turn your head from side to side. You will see where the light naturally falls onto your face.

'My number one tip for blush, whether it's cream or powder or liquid, is once you have applied it, go back over it with your foundation brush or beauty blender that you used for your base makeup. Sounds super simple, but by doing this you create blush that looks like it comes from within, rather than sitting on top of the skin; it also ensures the blend is seamless!'
HANNAH BENNETT, MAC SENIOR ARTIST

ESSENTIAL AREAS TO HIGHLIGHT

Cheekbones – start at the most common place where everyone focuses their highlighter. Applying product here will give the appearance of a natural lift. When applying you want to blend on top of your cheekbone and softly move up and around the outside of your eye area. Doing this will make sure there isn't a harsh line of highlighter.

Nose – you will see that light naturally hits the tip and bridge of your nose, so these will be the points where you add a touch of highlighter. I actually like to use my finger to dab a small amount on, which I find gives a natural finish.

Cupid's bow – light naturally falls onto your cupid's bow, the curved section at the top of your lip. Using my finger, I apply a small dab of highlighter there to define my lip shape.

Brow bone – I love highlighting my brow bone. I apply the highlighter with my finger or a small brush to give a lifted appearance.

Chin – another point on the face where light naturally hits. Apply highlighter to the centre of your chin, making sure to really blend it out so it looks natural.

Collarbones – I don't do this all the time, mainly in summer, but if I'm wearing a bandeau top or dress I love to add a touch of shimmer to my collarbones. It enhances your bone structure and just makes them pop.

Inner corner of the eyes – It's amazing what a small dot of highlighter can do when you strategically place it on the inner corner of your eyes. It widens your eyes, makes you look more awake and I find it finishes off your eye makeup look. How you place your inner-corner highlight will depend on what eye makeup you've gone for. For example, if I've just opted for a simple mascara look I will blend a small dot literally on my inner corner. However, if I've created an inner-corner eyeliner look I will add a line of highlight along the underneath of the eyeliner. When highlighting the inner corner of your eye you can either use a brush or a highlighting pencil.

FRECKLES

I want to start off by saying that freckles are beautiful. They're natural and they're a part of you! If you have freckles you might opt for minimal makeup to show off your natural beauty, but if you like a full-coverage look, be warned that they might get covered in the process. I have a great tip that can bring your freckles back and it's also great if you want to faux the freckle look. There's something about freckles for me; they make your skin look natural and healthy, and I use the fake freckle technique to disguise pimples! If you are going to try recreating

My top picks:
Affordable: *Makeup Revolution Freckle Me Pen*
Mid-range: *Freck Faux Freckle*

freckles or drawing them back in after applying makeup you should use a technique that makes them as natural-looking as possible. There are actually faux-freckle products on the market now, and some of them make it super-easy to create that look.

I've personally tried many ways to achieve a natural faux-freckle look and this one is by far the best that I've found. I use Benefit Cosmetics Brow Styler and choose the shade that's closest to my eyebrow colour. It's double-ended but you're going to take the powder end and shake it onto a makeup mixing palette or clean dry surface. What you will see is lots of different-sized speckles of powder. You then take your middle finger and gently tap on top of the speckles so you transfer them onto your finger. Then dab wherever you want your freckles to go. I tend to focus on my nose, cheeks and blending up to the forehead.

Keep repeating this process until you're happy with your freckle placement. I then like to go in with the powder applicator and enhance any beauty spots and add extra freckles. Once your freckles are all placed, grab your powder brush and tap powder over the top, pressing it into your skin. The freckles will slightly lighten in this process and the result will look super-natural.

'There are so many ways to create faux freckles but whatever way I do it I always apply a layer of bronzer onto the skin first (normally across the nose, cheeks and forehead). Freckles come out with the sun so warming up the base in the areas you will apply them helps them to look more natural.'
**HANNAH BENNETT,
MAC SENIOR ARTIST**

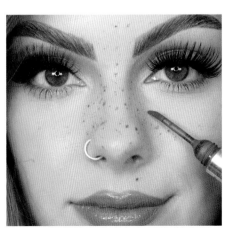
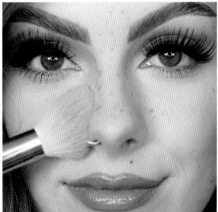

BROWS

When it comes to brows it's such a personal preference as to how you have them. I swear there is a new brow trend every week; one minute it's the bushy look, then it's slim brows, then everyone is having them laminated. Whatever the trend, find what works for you and your facial shape – it's amazing how eyebrows can completely transform your face.

My brows are something I've worked on a lot over the years and I've finally got to a place where I'm super-happy with them. Having a presence online means I put my face out there for the world to see daily and I've had a fair share of comments about my eyebrows. This definitely affected how I wore them, and I was always trying the latest trends for my brows to 'fit in', but I never liked any of them.

My natural brow hairs don't grow upwards, they grow sideways, which was something I struggled with for years until brow lamination came along. This innovative technique essentially smooths all your brow hairs while lifting and shaping them. It's a great alternative to microblading (see below)!

Lamination has given me the brows I've always wanted, and I don't think I'd ever steer away from this technique. My brows are now fuller and have really enhanced my face with a natural lift. And the great thing about lamination is that I can do it with an at-home kit. I use the Diablo Brow Lamination Kit which comes with an easy-to-follow step-by-step and all the products are labelled. It's a three-step application where you 'lift', 'fix' and 'nourish' your brows into their new lifted position. I laminate my brows every 3–4 months and it's made it a lot easier for me to do my brows every day. They look great with and without brow gel now.

But lamination is just one brow technique; there are many other options:

Microblading – this involves adding tiny brow-like strokes to your skin using a needle and pigment – kind of like a tattoo. It's semi-permanent and great for those who may have overplucked or who suffer from hair-loss conditions like alopecia. I got my brows microbladed once – I loved how they looked at the start, but when they healed it just didn't do anything for my brows and I've been left with red scarring from the pigment of this treatment. So if this is something you want to do, seriously consider the long-term implications of it.

Powder brows – also known as ombre brows, this treatment is similar to microblading in that a machine is used to deposit colour in between your brow hairs. Essentially it looks like you've applied brow powder, but this treatment lasts for 1–3 years. It fills in your brows, makes them look fuller and means you don't need to worry about them when it comes to applying your makeup.

Tinting – this process uses a semi-permanent brow dye in a tone that's close to the natural colour of your brow hair. This technique is great if you want fuller-looking brows and it'll help speed up your brow routine. Like hair dye, it's temporary, so as your brows grow and are exposed to the sun they will fade, which makes it a good option if you want to experiment with looks that won't have a permanent impact.

Threading – this technique has been around for years and involves using thin threads that are twisted in a way that gently plucks your hair out from the root. It's quick and a great way to shape your brows.

Waxing – another method of hair removal that shapes your brows and gets rid of unwanted hairs.

These are some of the main brow techniques, but you don't need to get a treatment done to be happy with your brows. You might love your natural brow shape and colour and a gel could be enough for you.

When you know what brow shape and style you love you need to find makeup products to help you achieve that look, such as brow gel (clear or coloured), pencils, fine-liner pens, powders and pomades. What style of brow you want to create will determine which products you choose. I use a gel to set my laminated brows in place – I like the Benefit 24-hour Brow Setter, which literally keeps my brow hairs in place ALL. DAY. LONG. It's by far the best brow gel I've used. When I set my hairs, I set them flat against my skin, and I do this before I start my base makeup and remove any excess gel around my brows. However, a brow gel can be used in whichever way works for you. You might prefer your brow hairs to be fluffier so just use a brow gel to comb them through and up. This can be done once your base makeup has been set.

If you want a more natural look when you fill in your brows, I'd opt for a pencil, powder or fine-line pen. You can build up the application and these give a softer finish. With a pencil you can shape the outer edge of your brow, or with an ultra-fine pencil or pen you can draw hair-like strokes that can blend in with your natural brow hair, making them appear fuller.

If you want a bolder brow look a pomade might be a better option. When using a pomade you need a really sharp-angled brow brush so that you can either block-fill your brows or use the brush to create hair-like strokes. I find a pomade works great if you're trying to achieve that ombre brow look, where you fill in the end of your brows and lightly fill in the start.

Once you've achieved your chosen brow shape and filled them in, apply concealer to the underneath edge of your brow to highlight and define the shape and make them pop.

Overall, try not to worry about trends too much, but there's no harm in experimenting – you never know, you might discover a new way of doing your brows that you prefer or that speeds up your brow routine.

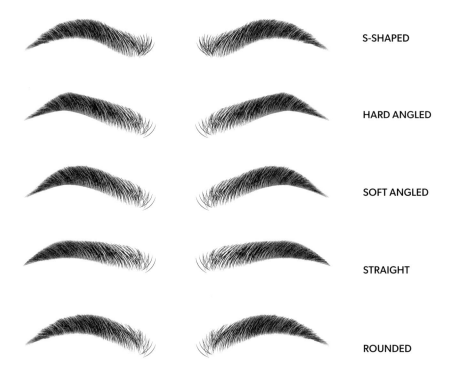

S-SHAPED

HARD ANGLED

SOFT ANGLED

STRAIGHT

ROUNDED

MY TOP PICKS

Brow pencil:
Affordable: Revolution Duo Brow Pencil
Mid-range: MAC Eyebrows Styler
High-end: Benefit Cosmetics Precisely, My Brow Pencil Ultra
Sustainable: Alkemilla Eco Bio Cosmetic Eyebrow Pencil

Pomade:
Affordable: Revolution Brow Pomade
Mid-range: NYX Professional Makeup Tame & Frame Tinted Brow Pomade
High-end: KVD Beauty Super Pomade Vegan Eyeliner
Sustainable: Ecobrow Defining Wax

Brow gel:
Affordable: NYX Professional Makeup Brow Glue
Mid-range: Lime Crime Bushy Brow Gel
High-end: Benefit Cosmetics 24-hour Brow Setter
Sustainable: Ecooking Eyebrow Gel

Fine liner:
Affordable: Barry M Cosmetics Feather Brow Defining Pen
Mid-range: NYX Professional Makeup Lift & Snatch! Brow Tint Pen
High-end: Anastasia Beverly Hills Brow Pen

Brow powder:
Affordable: Lottie London Brow Volume Powder
Mid-range: Sleek MakeUP Brow Kit
High-end: Benefit Cosmetics Brow Styler Eyebrow Pencil & Powder Duo
Sustainable: Lily Lolo Eyebrow Duo

EYE MAKEUP

Everyone will find a certain way of doing their own makeup that works for them and when it comes to eye makeup, I like to do this after my base makeup. However, some prefer doing this before their base and that's mainly because they don't need to worry about product dropping off makeup brushes onto their perfectly set foundation.

The reason I prefer doing my eye makeup after all the steps listed above, is that if I'm doing a wing liner look, for example, I have to carefully apply concealer and foundation around the edge of the liner, which makes it difficult to blend, and you can't apply eyeshadow under your bottom lid to finish off a look because you need to do that after concealer.

There are things you can do to help with eyeshadow fallout, though, the most obvious being don't load your brush up with too much product – pick up your eyeshadow onto your brush and give it a few taps to remove any excess, then build up your eyeshadow. This also makes blending easier. Or you could purchase eyeshadow shields; these disposable curved pads stick underneath your eye and catch the fallout. The downside to these is that they're sticky and can pull your base makeup off, so if you've opted for a full coverage base, don't stick them down, just hold them under your eye while you apply makeup with the other hand.

Another tip is to make sure your base is fully set with setting powder before doing your eye makeup. This will help in removing any fallout because the excess eyeshadow won't have any cream products to stick to, or you can blow the eyeshadow off your cheeks or grab a clean, fluffy powder brush and ever so lightly brush it away. This is what I tend to do and 99% of the time it works fine.

When it comes to eye makeup, you can be as creative or as simple as you like. Anything goes and I love that. I'm a super-creative person so if I have an occasion I or I'm going out for dinner I love to switch things up and try to create a different look each time, but for day-to-day life, I have a few core go-to looks that I choose between.

Everyday Eye-makeup Looks

Let's start with everyday eye-makeup looks. This is different for everyone – some of us might not wear makeup during the day and keep it just for occasions, while some of us might opt for something quick and easy as we like those extra minutes in bed. I personally like to mix between opting for either a full face look or something a bit lighter but eye makeup is a step I never miss.

Here are my go-to ways to do my everyday eye makeup.

ONLY MASCARA OR LASHES

A super-simple, quick and easily achievable look is keeping your eyelids bare and only wearing mascara or lashes. I love this; it helps draw attention to the eyes by opening them up and making them appear larger.

I like to mix and match between mascara or false lashes. Most of the time it depends on what I'm doing that day, so if I'm running errands I will opt for mascara, but if I want a more glammed-up look, I'll choose big false lashes.

When it comes to choosing a mascara, think about what your natural lash is like and what you want the mascara to do. Do you want length, volume, thickening or curling?

LASH LENGTHENING – a favourite of mine is the Maybelline Lash Sensational Sky High Mascara. It's got a flexible brush that bends to the natural shape of your lashes from root to tip, extending every single lash with the added synthetic fibres in the formula. This is great if you have short or sparse lashes, as the synthetic fibres in the formula bind to your natural lash and make them appear longer. If you are after a more sustainable formula without synthetic fibres, look for lengthening mascaras that have berry pigments, cocoa fibres or black tea.

> **My top picks:**
> **Affordable:** *Rimmel Extra Long Lash Mascara*
> **Mid-range:** *Maybelline The Falsies Instant Lash Lift Mascara*
> **High-end:** *Huda Beauty Legit Lashes*
> **Sustainable:** *NATorigin Lengthening Mascara*

THICKENING AND VOLUMISING – a volumising mascara is universal and works great on all lash lengths and density. My holy grail product is Too Faced's Better Than Sex mascara – the formula does everything, and it lasts all day long. It has fibres that bind to your lash to build that volume and length and the hourglass brush helps to curl.

My top picks:
Affordable: e.l.f. Volume Plumping Mascara
Mid-range: L'Oréal Paris Volume Million Lashes Mascara
High-end: Lancôme Lash Idôle Volumising Mascara
Sustainable: Gen See Spectator Sport Mascara

CURLING – if you find your lashes are quite straight and flat you'll love a curling mascara. I particularly love the Benefit Cosmetics Roller Lash. It curls and lifts your lashes from root to tip and the formula is designed to be long-lasting so your lashes won't flatten throughout the day. My favourite thing about this mascara is the 'Hook 'n' Roll' brush, which is great at grabbing each lash and separating, lifting and curling them individually. Expect longer-looking, curvier lashes with this one!

My top picks:
Affordable: Collection Max Curve Curling Mascara
Mid-range: Maybelline Colossal Curl Bounce Mascara
High-end: Dior Iconic Overcurl Mascara
Sustainable: INIKA Curvy Lash Mascara

LASH DEFINING – if you like the full-on fluttery lash look, a lash-defining mascara might be for you. These mascaras focus on combing through your lashes, separating them and making them clump-free. They also lengthen the lashes and add volume. I find mascaras with a rubber wand the best for separating lashes, like the Mac Cosmetics MACStack Mascara Mega Brush.

My top picks:
Affordable: Barry M Cosmetics Feature Length Mascara
Mid-range: KIKO Milano Ultra Tech + Volume and Definition Mascara
High-end: Charlotte Tilbury Pillow Talk Push Up Lashes! Mascara
Sustainable: ZAO Makeup Definition Mascara

WATERPROOF/SMUDGE-PROOF –

if your lashes are naturally long and when wearing mascara your lashes touch your skin when you look up or down, you might want to opt for a waterproof or a smudge-proof formula. You won't want black smudge marks around your eyes halfway through the day! Ditto if you're at the gym, you're somewhere hot or you're likely to shed a few tears. A lot of brands actually offer waterproof or smudge-proof versions of their lengthening, curling, lash-defining and volumising products, too.

My top picks:
Affordable: *MUA Eye Define Waterproof Mascara*
Mid-range: *L'Oréal Paris Paradise Waterproof Mascara*
High-end: *BADgal BANG! Waterproof Mascara*
Sustainable: *Ere Perez Avocado Waterproof Mascara*

When it comes to applying mascara, my top tip is to always use a lash curler first. They make a huge difference by giving your natural lash a curl and lift, then you can go straight in with your mascara. Doing this also means you won't need to layer your mascara. And if you're thinking 'are lash curlers damaging?', when used correctly, no, they're not! As long as you have a steady hand and don't tug on your lashes, and you clean the curlers between each use, you will be fine.

To create fuller-looking lashes, before you apply mascara take a little bit of eyeshadow, in the same colour as your eyebrow, and a small-angled brush, then apply it to your upper lash line on the eyelid. It can be very subtle, but this darkness will make your lashes look thicker and more voluminous once the mascara is applied.

If you want your lashes to look lifted and your eyes open but also don't want to look like you are wearing makeup, curl your lashes and try applying brown mascara only on the roots of your lashes (not the tips). This is a trick we use at fashion week a lot when the models need to look fresh and as if they just woke up looking perfect without any makeup!

'If you love the doe-eyed, 60s Twiggy lashes you can create the same effect in a natural way by using a thin brush and some gel eyeliner. Apply small dots under your bottom lash line between each lower lash to create the illusion that your bottom lashes are fuller. Your natural eyelashes fall over the dots, so you don't really see them, but the lashes look like they are thicker from the roots.'

**HANNAH BENNETT,
MAC SENIOR ARTIST**

More of a false-lash wearer? I love wearing false eyelashes on their own with no other eye makeup. There are so many different styles of these on the market, but the three that work well on their own have a super-thin, flexible lash band, individuals or falscara. Falscara by KISS is a new way to lash, where you apply a bond to your natural lash, apply wisps of lashes in small sections to the underneath of your top lash and seal them together. It's an amazing new kit if you love the look of lash extensions but don't want to deal with strip lashes.

Individual lashes are great if you're happy with how your own lashes look with mascara but maybe want to add a few on the outer edges for a lift or for volume. I tend to opt for strip lashes as I love to have the option of picking from multiple styles. When applying false lashes with no other eye makeup, I have the best technique to share – thanks to a TikTok viral hack that went around!

Step 1: Select your chosen false eyelashes, measure them up against your lash line and trim if needed. I trim the outer lash to make them shorter.

Step 2: Grab a makeup brush and wrap your false eyelashes around the handle. This will make sure there's a nice even bend in the lash band so they will shape to your eye more easily.

Step 3: Apply eyelash glue to the lash band – the application is key here: you're going to want to apply it like you normally would, but then also add a little along the top edge of the lash band, where the false eyelashes start to fan out.

Step 4: When the glue is tacky, apply the lash with pointed eyelash-specific tweezers to your lash line. I stick down the inner lash first, then the centre and work my way out. Squeeze the false eyelashes as close to your natural lash line as possible with the tweezers. Once your lash is in place, using your finger or lash tweezers, close your eye and press the skin on your eyelid on top of the lash band. It will adhere to the top of the false eyelashes; essentially you will have sandwiched your false eyelashes between your natural lash and the skin on your eyelid, creating a seamless finish. Your lashes will look flawless, natural and stay in place all day.

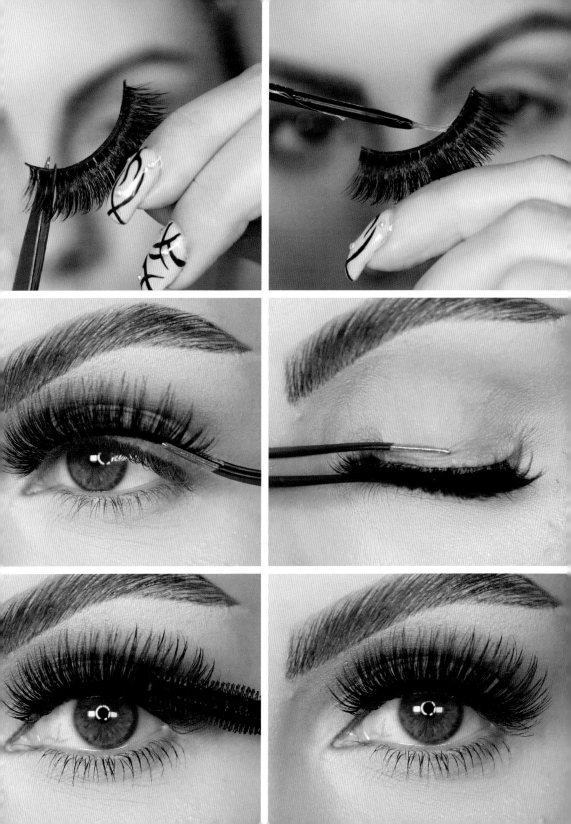

When I first tried that hack I couldn't believe I hadn't discovered it before. Your lashes look so natural and even when closing your eyes the adhesion is seamless. Oh, and I always apply mascara after my false strip-lash application. I find this works best as I can then blend my natural lashes into the false lashes.

WING EYELINER

Another one of my go-to everyday eye looks is liquid eyeliner, and I know this is the same for many others – it's a timeless classic that suits everyone when applied according to their eye shape. It enhances your eyes and can make a huge difference in shaping them and emphasising your lashes.

> **TOP TIP:**
> If you're like me and have allergies to lash glue, be careful which brand you use. Unfortunately, you're not going to know about an allergy until you try products, but if you're sensitive, maybe opt for a hypoallergenic eyelash glue at first that's latex-free – Duo have a great one. I sadly can't even use that so I opt for an eyelash adhesive that's acrylate-free – Tatti Lashes have a formula for super-sensitive eyes. Or you could try KISS Falscara range as the bond only goes on your lashes and not on your skin.

Mastering a wing liner look can be tricky, and being able to apply it the same way every day is even trickier. However, if you have the right tools you can achieve the perfect winged eyeliner. Don't be put off if you don't get it right the first time, you'll master it with a bit of practice.

First let's look at what wing eyeliner works for your eye shape:

Almond – having almond-shaped eyes means you can get away with a lot of different eyeliner styles, but a classic cat-eye wing works so well. Apply a thin line to the inner corner and make it thicker as you work your way to the end of your eye, then lift and wing it out to create a flick.

Deep-set – you don't want to weigh your eyes down too much with eyeliner here, so keep the focus for the liner on the outer section. Start applying a thin line in the centre of your eye to the outer corner, then make a short flick.

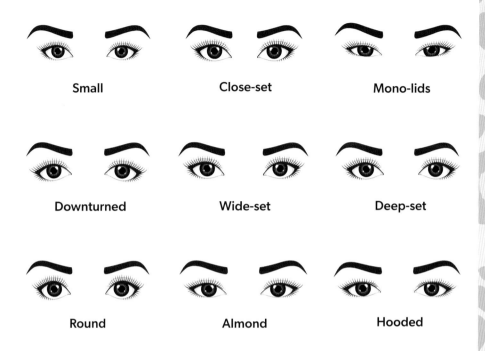

Small **Close-set** **Mono-lids**

Downturned **Wide-set** **Deep-set**

Round **Almond** **Hooded**

Mono-lids – since you can't see much of the eyelid you can make the liner across the top of your lash line as thick as you want and when it comes to the wing, exaggerate it and extend it out with a sharp flick. This will really elongate the eyes.

Downturned – if your outer corner drops lower than the inner corner, your eyes are downturned. When applying a wing you want to really lift it so it's angled towards your temples and keep it short, this will really accentuate your eye shape.

Wide-set – if the distance between your eyes is greater than the width of one eye from corner to corner, you have wide-set eyes. With a wing liner you're going to want to accentuate the inner corners of your eyes. You can do this by drawing your eyeliner past the end of the inner eye, following your eye shape and bringing the liner back in to join your lower lash line. Keep the liner the same thickness along your top lash liner and only do a small flick.

Close-set – if you have a small gap between your eyes, do the opposite to wide-set. You want to elongate your wing but keep the liner across your lash line thin.

Round – to balance your eye shape, focus on creating an elongated wing that can widen your eye. Create a thin line across your lash line with your eyeliner, thickening it from the centre to the outer corner into a sharp wing.

Hooded – if you find your lid crease covers your lid you'll want to draw your wing liner with your eyes looking forward. Start with the wing and mark out the bottom line following the angle of your waterline towards to the end of your brow tip. Keeping your eyes open, looking forward and relaxed, connect the end of your wing to the end of your eye crease. Still looking forward, make a dot on your lash line where you want your wing to start. Draw a thin line along your lash line and extend out towards the tip of the wing. You will end up with a box above the wing which you fill in. It'll look like a bat wing liner when your eyes are shut, but a seamless classic wing when your eyes are open.

Small – if you have small eyes try this application technique to really make them bold and pop. Apply a wing liner from the centre of your lid, keeping the line thin and consistent to the outer flick. Brighten your lower lash line with a white eyeliner and smudge black eyeshadow or kohl eyeliner under your lower lash line ending before you reach the centre of your eye.

My top picks:
Affordable: e.l.f. Cosmetics Precision Liquid Eyeliner
Mid-range: Urban Decay Perversion Fine Point Eye Pen
High-end: Code8 Precision Liquid Eyeliner
Sustainable: ZAO Liquid Eyeliner Refillable

Picking the right products is key when it comes to applying eyeliner. You want an eyeliner that is flexible and sharp to be able to create thin lines that you can build up into your chosen eyeliner style. Having concealer and a sharp-angled brow brush is useful too, to rectify any small mistakes. Personally, I find a liquid eyeliner with a felt-tip nib the best product to create a classic wing liner look, or use a gel eyeliner that comes in a pot and you apply with an eyeliner brush or a pencil eyeliner. However, I find a pencil eyeliner doesn't tend to last as long as liquid.

Another thing to think about is colour – will you pick black or brown? Both colours work great for everyday wear; black is sharper and sleeker whereas brown will give a softer look.

When applying eyeliner, be confident. A great tip is to map out where you want to draw your eyeliner by putting small dots along your lash line and wing. I use this hack all the time whenever I'm creating graphic liner looks. It also helps you when trying to match what you've done on one eye with the other.

On the days I opt for a winged liner look I also like to add a neutral colour in the crease. This won't work for every eye shape, but I find on my almond-shaped eyes

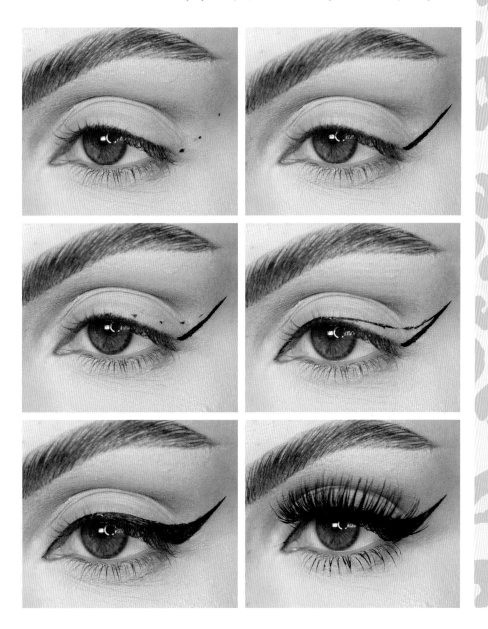

it makes my eyes pop. I do this with either bronzer or a warm brown shade to add depth to my overall eye look.

Lashes are the finishing touch to any wing liner look and either mascara or false strip lashes work great. I tend to prefer false strip lashes as I find the placement of these can enhance your elongated eye shape even more. Instead of applying your false lashes along your lash line, glue them down along the pathway of your liquid eyeliner, lifting out at the wing.

NEUTRAL EYESHADOW

My final go-to everyday look is a neutral shadow – think earthy nudes and browns. I like to select just one colour and buff it out all over my lid, then blend out towards my temples. This paired with a wing eyeliner looks great, or I just opt for mascara with false strip lashes. Super-simple, super-easy and such a wearable everyday look.

I tend to stick to matte eyeshadows when I create this look, but you could definitely switch things up and opt for a metallic shimmer on the lid or even a pop of highlight on the inner corner. This is a simple eye look that you could wear to work then for after-work drinks, quickly jazzed up in the bathroom before you head out.

In summer, instead of opting for a neutral eyeshadow, pick a colour that maybe matches the outfit that you're wearing or complements your eye colour.

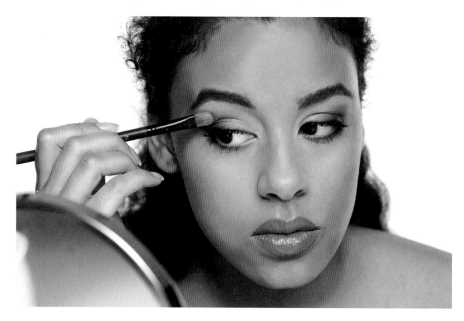

Experimenting With Colour

Oh, what fun you can have experimenting with colour. The possibilities are endless! Coloured eyeshadows, eyeliners, even mascara. It can be a little bit overwhelming with the amount of choice on the market and numerous ways in which you can wear colourful makeup, but I have a few go-to options I love and want to share with you all – especially if you tend to steer away from this approach.

Even though I believe that everyone can and should be able to wear every colour, some shades do tend to suit certain skin tones and eye colours more than others; then there's the issue of applying it, so it's blended well. I can understand why a lot of people shy away from it.

WHAT COLOURS YOU SHOULD WEAR BASED ON YOUR EYE COLOUR

This is a rule I personally never follow. I love experimenting with makeup, and I will wear every colour of the rainbow – either on their own or all together. I think as long as you love the makeup look you've created you will naturally ooze confidence and it'll look fabulous on you.

However, if you're looking to add colour into your makeup looks and it's something you've never tried before, find out which ones suit your eye colour, as you're kind of guaranteed that they will suit you.

COLOUR EYESHADOWS FOR EYE COLOURS:

Green eyes	rose gold, pink, purple, plum, bronze, silver
Blue eyes	orange, warm brown, copper, gold
Hazel eyes	pink, purple, copper, gold, green
Brown eyes	gold, purple, bronze, teal, silver, rose gold, emerald green, cobalt blue, burgundy
Grey eyes	blue, green, grey, silver, earthy neutrals, maroon

Eye Looks

Let's start with how to add colour into your eye makeup. If you're new to this, I have lots of ways that you can introduce colour subtly. But I also have lots of ideas for when you feel confident to explore bolder looks.

COLOUR MASCARA

Who remembers when blue mascara was a thing? I'm obsessed with a colour mascara. It instantly makes your eyes pop and just adds a touch of playfulness to your look. You can pretty much find any colour of mascara now, so have a play around, wear one colour on its own or even combine two or more! I find when you've gone bold with your mascara you should pair it with a nude lip, as you don't want to take the focus away from your colourful lashes.

COLOUR EYELINER

If colour mascara is a little too much for you, try switching up your eyeliner instead. There are so many ways you can combine colour into an eyeliner look and here are just some of my favourites.

Dots – if you've never tried colour before, start with dots. You can be as experimental as you like with this technique. Try creating your usual wing eyeliner look and finish it off with a coloured liquid eyeliner, maybe one that complements your outfit, and draw a small dot under your eye, in the centre. If you don't like a wing liner look, try the same dot but paired with mascara. Then when you're ready to introduce more colour, add more dots! What I love about this technique is anything goes. Apply the dots wherever you want; apply one dot on the inner corner of your eye and three dots where you would draw your wing, or apply a few dots on the inner of your eye but following your eye shape. Have fun with it and get your creative juices flowing.

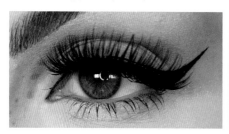
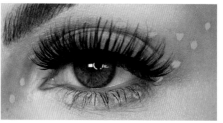

Waterline and undereye – if you're a wing eyeliner wearer you could experiment with colour by adding it into your waterline – the line of skin between the eyelashes and the eye – paired with your wing liner. You will want a super-pigmented, waterproof pencil eyeliner for this and you can go as bright or pastel as you want with the shade. Then when you want to intensify and increase the colour, you can extend it out past your waterline and smudge it under your lower lash line until it meets the end of your wing.

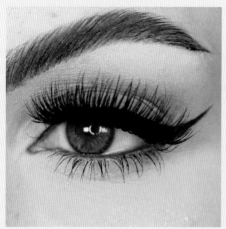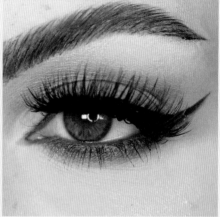

On top of your wing liner – another option is to grab a coloured liquid eyeliner and draw a thin line following the outer edge of your go-to wing liner look. Or if you want to amplify your wing even more, switch out your black/brown liquid liner and create your go-to wing liner look with a colour instead.

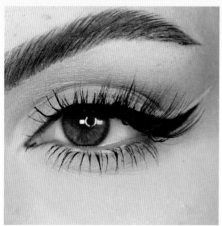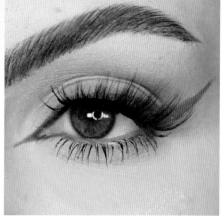

Graphic liner looks – if you want to get even more experimental with your eyeliner, try different liner looks using a coloured eyeliner. For example, the floating eyeliner trend – this is where you draw a line above the crease of your lid, following your eye shape, in the section between your lid and brow bone. If you want to, connect the end of that line to the end of a wing liner for a different look entirely. Or apply a coloured wing liner and find an eye pencil in the same shade to go into your waterline and under the lower lash line, creating a bold one-coloured look. You could even try out one of my favourites, a reverse winged liner, where the eyeliner is on your lower lash line instead of the upper.

Once you've experimented with applying one colour, if you're wanting to go even bolder you could use two or three shades. Try creating an ombre wing liner by blending a few shades of eyeliners together, or try the floating eyeliner trend with two coloured lines instead of one.

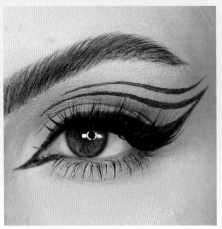 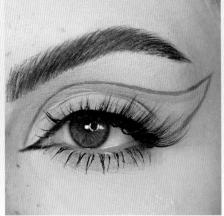

EYESHADOW

Let's move on to eyeshadow, as this is where you get to have even more fun. If you're new to wearing coloured eyeshadow there are plenty of ways you can include it in your makeup looks subtly, before you try something bold.

There are three types of eyeshadow formula on the market: cream, liquid and powder.

Cream – these tend to have a long wear and don't crease when blended. They're super-easy to apply with your finger or a brush and you'll find them in matte or shimmer shades. A cream eyeshadow makes a good base for your powder eyeshadows. For example, if you want to create a pastel eye look with a pale pink eyeshadow, pop on a white cream shadow base under the powder eyeshadow and it'll make it pop and appear true to colour.

Liquid – super-lightweight, easy to blend and can be applied in one coat. Liquid eyeshadows are also very buildable, so if you want a rich colour you can apply a few coats. These are long-lasting and if you want to add a shimmer or glitter to your makeup look, a liquid formula means you don't get any product fallout.

Powder – the formula that everyone knows, a powder eyeshadow. You can find these eyeshadows either pressed or loose. Pressed eyeshadow are the ones you find in palettes; they're super-pigmented, buildable and easy to blend. Using a pressed eyeshadow means you can blend a few colours into each other to create depth or even an ombre look.

Pressed eyeshadows have been formulated with a wetting agent, which is what keeps them moulded into pans. Loose pigments don't have this, meaning they have fewer ingredients in the formula and are much more lightweight. When using a loose-pigment eyeshadow, apply with a flat brush, making sure to tap any excess off the brush. You want to pack the colour on then switch to a fluffy brush to blur any harsh lines. Loose eyeshadows are so versatile, you can turn them into eyeliners by using a mixing liquid.

Before you start applying any eyeshadow on your lid you should prime similar to what you would do before applying base makeup (see page 24). An eye primer is great as it improves your eye texture, making makeup application smoother, longer-lasting and less likely to crease throughout the day. And if you're wearing a glittery or shimmer formula, use a glitter primer to really make the pigment pop.

For powder and shimmer eyeshadows, a great tip is to spritz your brush beforehand with setting spray then pack on the eyeshadow and apply. It'll make your powder eyeshadow into a metallic creamy wash that will glide across your lid. This is a game changer!

My top eye primers:
Affordable: e.l.f. Shadow Lock Eye Primer
Mid-range: Urban Decay Eyeshadow Primer Potion

Let me take you through some subtle ways of adding coloured eyeshadow into your eye looks.

Inner corner – the perfect look to start introducing yourself to colour. Pick an eyeshadow shade that either matches your outfit or complements your eye colour. Use a small round brush for this as it'll sit neatly into your inner corner, you could also use your little finger for this, but if you have long nails, go for the brush option. Start with a small amount of eyeshadow on your brush and tap the product to the inner corner of your eyes, then blend this as much as you want, focusing it around the shape of the inner eye. This looks great paired with mascara, false lashes or even a wing liner.

Wing liner and pop of colour – if you want to try something bold, why not jazz up your go-to wing liner by applying a colour eyeshadow to the underneath of your eye? Apply from your inner corner along your lower lashes and end on the outer corner of your eye. Use a small flat eyeshadow brush for this as it'll fit nicely under your lash line, then use a blending brush to buff the edge of the eyeshadow out. Finally, either apply a kohl eyeliner to your waterline in the same shade as the eyeshadow, or in black or white. This will tie the whole eye look together.

Eyeshadow colour – a simple look that's amazing paired with mascara or even false lashes is popping one single eyeshadow colour onto your eyelid. The key is blending the colour on your lid, into the crease and upwards towards your brow. If you're new to colour, why not try this look with a pastel eyeshadow first, then increase the pigment the more comfortable you feel. Or experiment with a metallic shade.

If this is an eye makeup look you love, you could switch things up and instead of blending the colour out upwards to your brow bone, give your look a 60s twist by keeping things sharp. Wing out your colour, then connect the end of your wing to the inner corner of your eye by drawing a line, following your eye shape, above your crease. Fill that shape with your chosen colour. Bold and dramatic! You could even outline the shape with a black liquid eyeliner to make it really pop.

To pack even more colour onto your eyes you can extend your one-colour eyeshadow under your lower lash line as well, so it's around your whole eye.

These are all great ways to introduce colour into your eye makeup looks. Start off trying lighter shades, then work your way up to more pigmented colours. Experiment and see which tones you prefer wearing, or match your makeup to your outfit or even hair colour to tie a look together. It gives you a good starting point if you're unsure about what colour to pick.

And if you're ready to go bold? Have fun! Mix and match a few shades together, maybe apply one colour to your lid and another under your lower lash line. Use multiple colours of eyeliners, draw shapes, use the dotting eyeliner technique. Get your creative juices flowing. And if you're stuck for inspiration, social media is a great place to look (TikTok, Pinterest, Instagram), but also look at magazines, books, nature, or sift through your wardrobe and get inspired by a print from a top or dress. Nothing is ever 'too much' when it comes to makeup. If you love it, wear it. People will feel the confidence oozing out of you!

EYE MAKEUP TECHNIQUES

When I have a bit of extra time to get ready, I like to spend a little longer on my eye makeup and use particular techniques to create a look. Some of these looks take practice, but if you use the right brushes, you'll get the knack in no time.

SMOKY EYE

Let's start off with a classic – the smoky eye. There are lots of different ways to create this iconic style, so it can be a little overwhelming knowing where to start. I've broken down this technique into a few simple steps.

- Apply an eye primer to the eye area.

- Blend a mid- to deep eyeshadow all over your lid, into your crease and upwards towards your brow. Take this shade as high as you want, but make sure you leave space below the brow.

- Take this shade along the underneath of your lower lash line as well.

- Apply a cream or liquid eyeshadow or even a creamy kohl eyeliner in a darker shade than you've just used along your lid lash line and blend upwards to your crease. Using this type of product tends to add an intense depth to the look, but you can use a powder eyeshadow if you prefer.

'Smoky eyes means something different to everybody, as a makeup artist I think it's really about the technique of blending. When I think of smoky eye, I automatically think of the 1920s, where buffed-out charcoal blacks were used all over the lid to give a kind of sexy, dream-like look to the eye. But a smoky eye to some people can also be just a little bit of dark-brown pencil smudged into the lash line. You can really make it as simple or as complicated as you want!

A great way to add some colour into your makeup is to add a metallic purple, green or blue on top of a black smoky eye. This is less intense than full colourful eye makeup, but when you layer a metallic shade on a black base the colour still pops. I also love a lived-in smoky eye – add some gloss or Vaseline on top of a black eye kohl with your finger, you don't need to add much because the product will move itself and create a gorgeous 90s grunge effect across the lid.'

**HANNAH BENNETT,
MAC SENIOR ARTIST**

Black tends to be the most common shade, but a dark grey or brown works well too. You want this shade to transition into the mid shade you applied first. If you've used a cream or liquid eyeshadow, take a similar shade in a powder form and tap it over the top – this will intensify the shade. When I create a smoky eye look I want the black to be super-pigmented.

> **My top picks:**
> **Affordable:** Rimmel London HD 5 Pan Eyeshadow
> **Mid-range:** Urban Decay Naked Basics 2
> **High-end:** Charlotte Tilbury The Rock Chick Luxury Palette
> **Sustainable:** Nicmac Beauty Refillable Eyeshadow Palette

- Take a kohl eyeliner in the same shade and line your waterline for maximum impact.

- Apply mascara or lashes and you're set!

Once you've mastered the basic steps to create a smoky eye, you can experiment with switching up the hue. Try a bronzed smoky eye, or even a royal blue. And if you want to make things a little easier, there are so many eye palettes on the market that can help you achieve this look instantly.

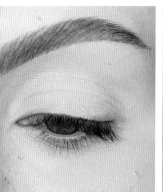
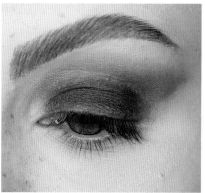
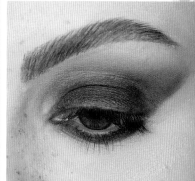
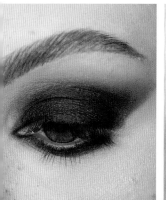
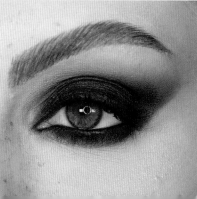
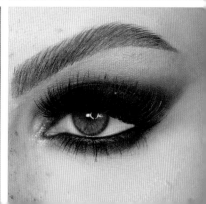

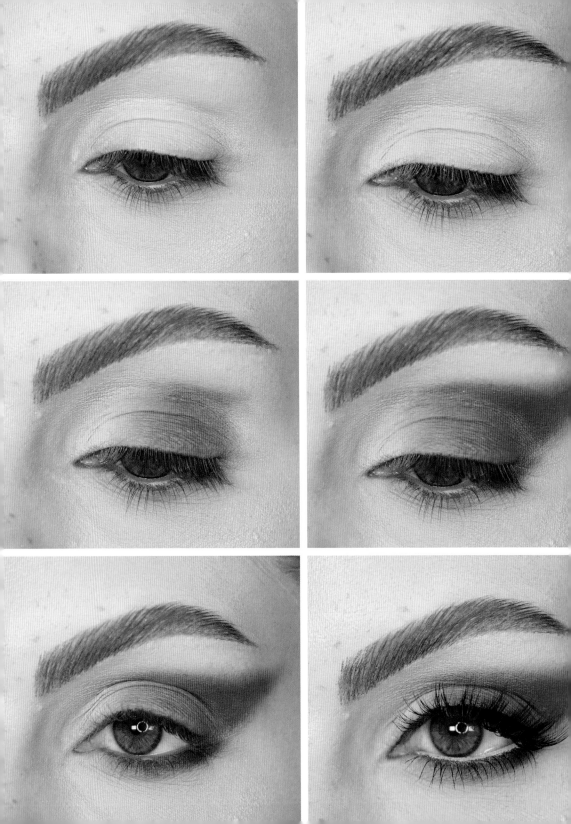

GRADIENT EYE MAKEUP

This is where the colours blend seamlessly from light to dark. They're dramatic and fun and you can use endless colour combinations. The key is all in the blending, so picking the right brushes is crucial to achieve a seamless gradient.

- Apply an eye primer to the eye area.

- Select your colour palette, you want to pick out 3–4 shades that go from light to dark. I use a powder eyeshadow for this as they blend well into one another.

- Start by selecting whichever colour is the lightest from your chosen shades. Apply this on the inner corner of your eye, blending upwards in a circular motion. Make sure the colour is more pigmented to the inner corner, and as you move outwards the colour will fade ready to blend into a new colour.

- Take your next shade for the gradient and tap that onto your lid just before the centre of your eye. Use a tapping motion so the colour is concentrated, then take a small and clean fluffy blending brush, blend slightly over the first colour in mini circular motions so they diffuse into one another.

- Then do the same again with your next shade. Apply to the other side of the centre of your lid, using the tapping method to concentrate the colour and then a small fluffy blending brush to melt into the previous colour. Repeat this as you work along your whole lid.

- You want to follow the shape of your eye when applying the shadow and leave a gap just below your brow.

- Once I've achieved the gradient on the top of my eye, I take the same colours and do the same on the underneath of my eye.

- It's totally up to you whether you add a liquid wing liner and lashes. Oh, and don't forget to add a kohl eyeliner to your waterline – this could be in white to brighten, or black to add drama or pick a shade the same as your deepest eyeshadow colour.

Once you've mastered a gradient eye you can experiment with multiple colours, keeping it monochromatic or combining matte and shimmer finishes.

CUT CREASE

I love a cut-crease eye makeup look. It creates the illusion of depth and widens your eyes. It also adds extra space on your lid so you can really showcase your chosen eyeshadow. When you get that crease sharp, oh does it feel good!

There are two ways you can create a cut crease – you can cut it along your whole eye or halfway. With this technique, essentially you apply a deeper eyeshadow above the natural crease of your eye, extending upwards towards your brow, then carve a defined line just above your natural crease using a concealer and apply a lighter shade to your lid. It creates a dramatic contrast and your eyes look super-defined. Let me take you through step by step:

- Apply an eye primer to the eye area.

- Select your chosen colour palette for the eye look. Apply a deep shade above your crease, packing it on just above where you want to 'cut'.

- Use a small blending brush to blend this upwards towards the brow bone. I like to take a slightly lighter shade in the same hue to help achieve a seamless blend.

- Once you're happy with the depth you've added above your crease, take an eyeshadow cut crease brush – this is a flat, dense, curved brush that's going to help you achieve that defined 'cut' line.

- Apply concealer to the brush and start carving your cut crease, following your natural crease shape. I like to look forwards when I'm doing this, so my cut crease is above the natural fold in my lid. You can cut your crease as high or as low as you want, depending on the look you want to achieve; there's no right or wrong way.

- If you're going to do a full cut crease, take the defined line out and wing the shape so it curves down to the outer eye and then lifts towards your brow tail/temple.

- For a half-cut crease, take the defined line above three-quarters of the way along your crease.

- Pack concealer over your whole lid to define the shape you cut for a full cut crease and for a half, apply to half of your lid.

- Select your chosen lid colour – this will be a lighter eyeshadow or maybe a shimmer or glitter pigment.

- For a full cut crease, apply this over your whole lid and wing it out. For a half cut crease, apply to the start of your lid and blend as you make your way to your outer eye. Switch back to your deep eyeshadow shade, apply this on the outer eye and blend inwards into your chosen lighter shade.

- Tie the look together with a kohl liner in your waterline.

- You can finish off with applying your mid and deep shades under your lower lash line and then a liquid wing liner, mascara or false lashes. Or all three!

One you've mastered a full and half cut crease there are so many other ways you can use this technique to create eye makeup looks. You could add in multiple shades to your lid and above the cut, all blending into each other to create a really colourful look. You could add a white, colour or glitter liquid liner along the cut crease line you've created to define it even more. Or add a touch of *Euphoria* to the look with eye gems along the crease. Or even try out a double cut crease – yes, a double! This is where you have a small gap between your lid shade and your deeper shade above the crease, where both edges are defined.

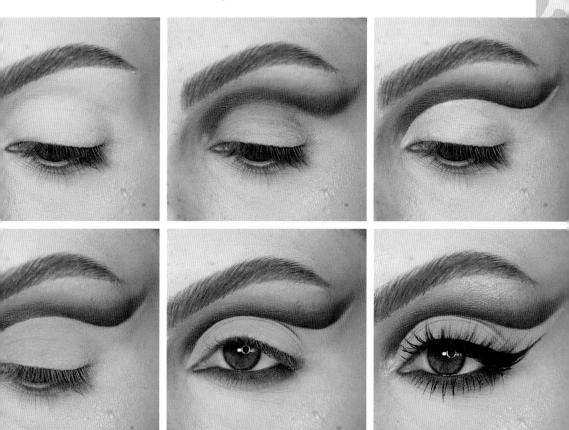

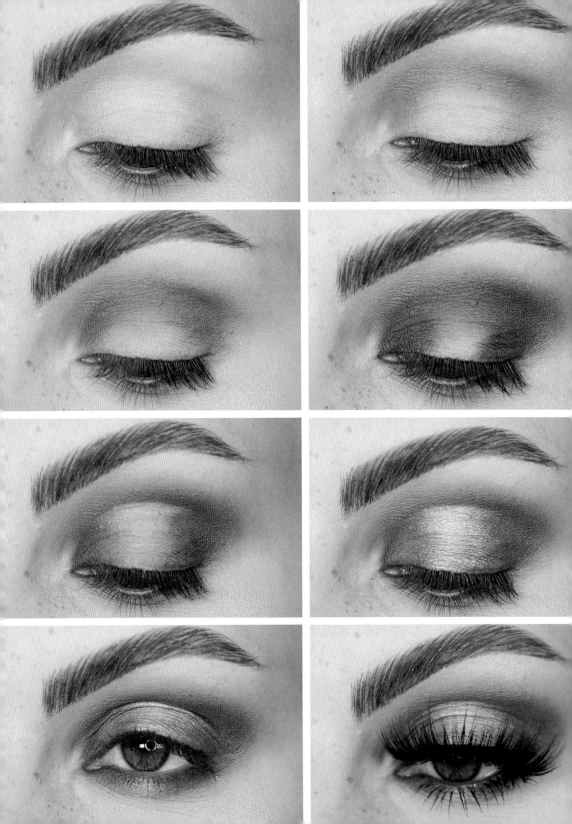

SPOTLIGHT OR HALO EYE MAKEUP

Another great eye makeup technique to try out is a spotlight or halo eye, where you place a light colour in the centre, in between a deeper shade on the outer and inner of your lid. This brings the light to the centre of the eyes, making them pop and appear rounder and wider. You can play around with so many colours to create this look, even different eyeshadow finishes and pigments.

- Apply an eye primer to the eye area.

- Select your colour palette – this could be neutral or bright.

- Apply a transition colour to your crease and blend upwards towards your brow and around your eye. This will be a lighter shade in the same hue as the deep colour you've selected.

- Apply a mid hue of that same shade into your crease to intensify the colour.

- Go in with your deepest shade and apply to the inner and outer of your lid and top of the crease in the centre of your eye. Avoid the centre of your lid area.

- I like to take my cut crease brush here, then apply concealer to the centre of the lid, patting it on and creating a curved defined edge along my crease at the top. You can either do this, or instead of defining your crease, blend the concealer in a straight line up, towards the centre of your brow.

- Then take your light eyeshadow – for this type of technique a metallic, shimmer or glitter shade works well, but you can use a matte hue. Pat this over the top of where you've applied your concealer.

- Blend the edges of this shade into your deep shade. Use a small fluffy brush to achieve a seamless blend.

- Replicate this under your lower lash line – apply the deep shade to the outer and inner sections, and in the centre apply your light shade, then blend these.

- Tie the look together with a kohl liner in your waterline.

- Finish with mascara or lashes.

Lips

Lips, for me, is the final step of a makeup look. My go-to lip shade tends to be a nude, but it does totally depend on what eye makeup I've picked. Lip colour and formula is something that's so personal, especially with there being an array of lipstick finishes on the market, from matte to gloss.

My top lipstick brands:
Affordable: *NYX Cosmetics*
Mid-range: *KVD Beauty*
High-end: *Code8 Beauty*
Sustainable: *Axiology*

A GUIDE TO LIPSTICKS

Lip stain/tints – a low-maintenance option, lipstick stains and tints last throughout the day and look natural. The only downside is they can be drying, so apply a balm first to moisturise your lips.

Lip crayon – easy to apply, smooth and a good mix between a balm/gloss and lipstick. Most lip crayons have been infused with moisturising ingredients, which is a great added benefit.

Lip gloss – Thankfully lip glosses have come a long way since the day where the wind would blow and stick your hair to your lips! A gloss formula now keeps your lips soft, shiny and chap-free.

Liquid lip – a formula I'm so grateful for – what did we do before liquid lipstick? They're super-pigmented, they look like a cream but dry matte, depending on which finish you opt for. There's no need to reapply as the formula is so long-wearing and they're smudge-free.

Matte – comes in the form of a bullet or a liquid lipstick. Super-pigmented and long-lasting, it leaves your lips with a flat matte finish. The only downside is a matte lip can be drying because they're made with less oil, so if you find your lips suffer when wearing a matte, pop a balm underneath to moisturise.

Creamy – a creamy finish, full coverage and pigmented. They slide on and keep your lips soft and hydrated.

Satin – somewhere in between a matte and cream lipstick, you'll find a satin lipstick soft and moisturising. With this type of lipstick you do tend to need to reapply throughout the day, but they could be a great option if your lips suffer with dryness.

Lip balm – available with a colour tint or clear. They are great for every day, worn under matte lipsticks, and are really hydrating.

Lip liners – small, lightweight and long-lasting, I love a lip liner! They help to define your lip shape and prevent lipstick bleeding. I apply a lip liner in a slightly darker shade than my chosen lipstick colour and sometimes, if I'm after a natural look, I find a lip liner close to my natural lip colour, line my lips, buff out and apply a gloss or balm to finish. A lip liner is so versatile.

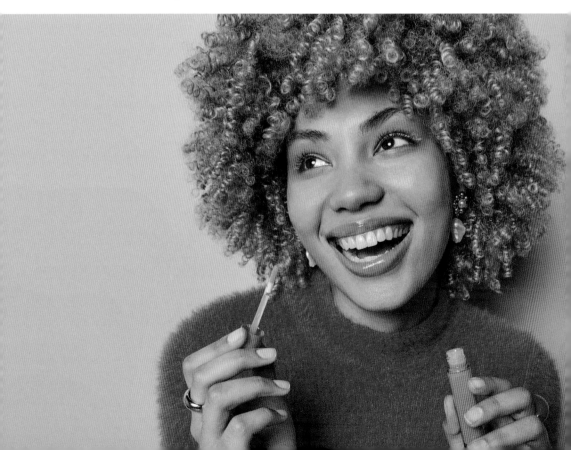

Once you've figured out which formula and finish of a lipstick you prefer, you need to find the right shade. This can be tricky with so many colours on offer, especially if you're trying to find the perfect red or nude lipstick. But this is where knowing your skin tone and undertones comes in handy.

When looking for a lip colour, find ones that will work for your undertone. For example, if you're after a red lipstick (which is a great way to add colour to a makeup look as it's timeless, classic and suits everyone), look for a red with the undertone that will suit you. Remember, undertones and skin tones are different (see page 32).

LIP COLOURS FOR UNDERTONES

Cool	lip colours with blue/purple undertones
Warm	lip colours with red/orange/brown undertones
Neutral	most hues work well

LIP COLOURS FOR SKIN TONE

Light/fair	light pinks, corals, nudes and beige
Medium	medium pinks, berry shades
Dark skin	browns, purples and deep reds

Ultimately, undertones, skin tones and eye colour will help guide you when picking colours, but they don't have to be followed. Try different shades and choose what you feel looks best on you and complements the overall makeup look you're trying to achieve.

Taking Off Makeup

You've worn your makeup all day long, your PJs are on and you're ready to hit the pillow. I think we've all been there where we've skipped taking off our makeup before bed. One night won't really make a difference to our skin, but if we constantly skip our evening cleanse and skincare routine, we're welcoming bacteria, clogged pores, breakouts and blackheads. Removing your makeup every night is a skincare must!

HOW TO REMOVE MAKEUP

First thing to do is pull your hair out of your face; you don't want to miss removing makeup along your hairline. Do this step and look cute using a cloth headband – you can find some adorable designs with bows and bunny ears.

Then remove your eye makeup. The eye area, as we all know, is delicate and can be sensitive, so find an eye-specific makeup remover with a gentle formula. The key to removing eye makeup is 'soaking' not 'rubbing'. Apply your remover to a reusable cotton pad and place it over your eye like you would a cucumber slice. Gently press down over your eye and hold it there for around 15–30 seconds. Your eye makeup should melt off, but if needed you can repeat this step. If there's any stubborn mascara or lash glue still left, soak a cotton bud in the same remover and use this along your lash line. Try to choose an eco-friendly cotton bud which has a bamboo stick rather than plastic. Ultimately, you need to find a good remover where you don't need to rub to get your eye makeup off.

Once your eye makeup is off, it's time to go in with a double cleanse. You want to remove your makeup then clean your pores to remove excess oils. Find a cleanser to suit your skin needs – this could be a micellar water, a cleansing oil or a foam cleanser. Micellar waters are great at removing makeup, but you want a cleansing oil, cream or balm product for your second cleanse.

I find the best way to use a cleanser is to wet your hands and apply the cleanser straight onto your face, then use your hands to massage it in. Splash warm water onto your face as you go to really break down the makeup. I like to grab a damp reusable makeup wipe and gently wipe my face so I know all of the makeup has been removed. Then I go in with a second cleanse to really make sure my skin is free of makeup and dirt. Don't forget to focus on areas like under your chin and neck, around the creases of the nose and your hairline. Pat your face dry with a clean flannel, then you're ready to follow up with your evening skincare routine – moisturiser, toner, serums.

If you have dry or sensitive skin, focus your cleansing routine to the evenings, then in the morning, before going in with your skincare and makeup products again, just splash your face with warm water. Washing your face twice a day works for most of us with combination, oily or acne-prone skin if we're using a gentle cleanser, but it can be irritating for dry or sensitive skin types. You don't need to wash your face twice a day; you shouldn't be washing it more than twice a day either. Work your routine around you and your skin. At the end of the day, you know your skin type the best.

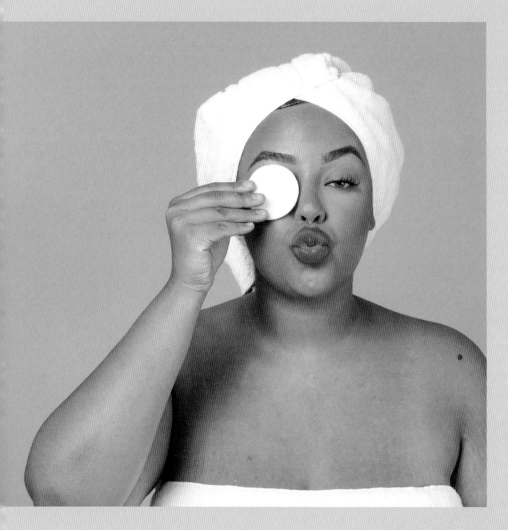

Makeup For Occasions

I don't know about you but doing my makeup for an occasion is an excuse for me to get glammed up. It's my chance to try out something new and get creative. We all have a go-to way for how we wear our everyday makeup, but when it comes to getting ready for an occasion, this is where we can switch things up and try out that cut crease technique or experiment with colour. Whether you're a minimalist or a maximalist I've got you sorted when it comes to your next event, date night or party.

Party Makeup

You're going out out. Whether that's a restaurant date night, clubbing with friends, a family party or it's the holidays and New Year; we all want to get glammed up, feel confident and look our best. Your outfit is sorted and it's time to figure out what makeup you're going to pair with it.

When I think about party makeup, I think glam, jewel tones, statement red lip, eye gems and glitter. Think about what the occasion is and what your outfit looks like. Are you wearing a little black dress, for example? A winged liner and a statement red lip could look incredible. Or maybe you're wearing a silver sequin dress and want to add a matching sparkle to your eye makeup with silver glitter lids. Maybe it's the holidays and you want to theme your look with festive golds, reds and greens. The getting ready part of the night is just as fun as the actual night itself if you ask me!

I've got four classic makeup looks to give you inspiration the next time you're getting glammed up. They're ideas that you can use as a bit of a starting point, then why not switch up the colours the next time?

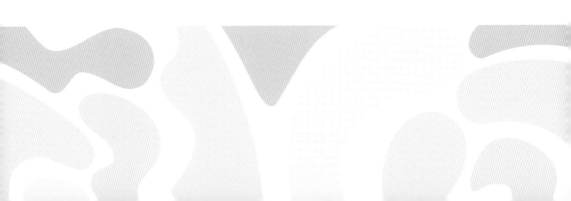

GLITTER LIDS

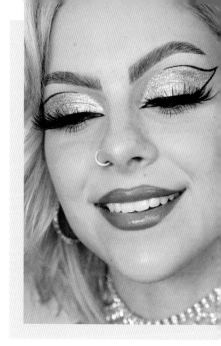

I don't need much of an excuse to wear glitter. I am obsessed with adding a sparkle to my makeup in any way that I can. Glitter lids is a great look for a party, especially in the lead up to the holidays. Glitter eyeshadows come in many forms – creams, powders, liquids and loose. I like to use a combination (see page 93 for a top tip for removing glitter!).

- Apply your base makeup, brows and prime the eye area.

- Apply a silver metallic liquid eyeshadow over the lid, defining the outer edge and winging it out.

- Apply a glitter primer over the top.

- Apply a silver, fine, loose glitter pigment – look for one that's eco-friendly to help the environment. EcoStardust is a brand I purchase from as they sell BioGlitter® – glitter that has been formed from natural and plant-derived polymer material that's been tested and proven to biodegrade into harmless substances in the natural environment.

- Apply with a brush, dampen it slightly with setting spray before dipping it into the glitter, as this will help pick up the pigment. Then apply using a tapping motion, to really pack it on the lid. Be careful of fallout, tap the brush to remove any excess glitter before applying or you could use an eyeshadow shield to help. If you do get fallout, use a clean, fluffy powder brush to buff off any speckles from your base makeup.

- Once you're happy with your glitter application, apply a winged liner across your lash line and follow the shape of where you've applied the glitter.

- Add a kohl eyeliner to your waterline and either mascara or false lashes to finish.

- Pair with a nude lipstick of choice.

BOLD LIPS - RED OR DARK PURPLE

Make your pout pop and your eyes fierce! I love pairing a deep-red or purple-hued lip with a sharp, dramatic winged liner. A red lip can look classic, but a purple lip can give you an edge. Both are great options for a party look, depending on your outfit and style.

- Apply your base makeup, brows and prime the eye area.

- Add depth into your crease using a mid dark neutral matte eyeshadow.

- Apply liner across your lash line and wing it out as far as you like. You're also going to wing out from your inner corner.

- Add a kohl eyeliner to your waterline and either mascara or false lashes to finish the eyes.

Choose either a deep red or purple hue and your chosen finish – satin, matte, gloss? I personally love a matte lipstick when I go out as I find them long-lasting and I tend to use a liquid lipstick formula. Line your lip in a similar tone and apply your chosen lipstick. If your lips are dry, add a balm under your liquid lip beforehand.

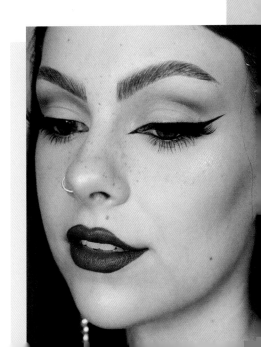

EYE GEMS

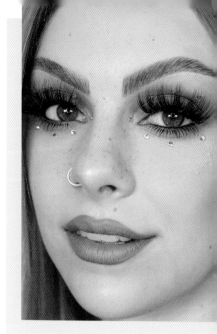

Since *Euphoria* trended, makeup looks with eye gems have popped up everywhere and they're great for a party look. They're super-quick to apply and can instantly give glam and sparkle to a simple, minimal makeup look. There are so many different ways you can incorporate eye gems; you could pair with a winged liner, apply them all over your lids, in different patterns across your eyes or with a coloured eyeshadow. You can keep the gems minimal or go all out.

You'll want flatback gems for this look. I like to buy mini boxes of different-sized gems from Amazon that come with a wax gem applicator – honestly the best tool, it makes it so easy to pick them up and the whole application process quick and easy. With flatback gems you will need to use eyelash glue to adhere them, or find ones that come as a sticker. That way you can just go ahead and stick them within your eye looks. Eye gems come in so many different colour variations, but I always steer towards using silver or holographic ones as these look great paired with silver jewellery.

- Apply your base makeup and brows and prime the eye area.

- Apply a white cream eyeshadow and buff it all over your lid.

- Choose an eyeshadow colour that matches your outfit, apply all over your lid into your crease and diffuse up towards your brow, making sure you leave space just below your brow bone. Then apply to the underneath of your lower lash line.

- Add a kohl eyeliner to your waterline, then finish with mascara or false lashes.

- Apply eye gems around the outer of your eye, in a circular shape, spreading them out easily. Start with the centre points of your eye to keep things symmetrical.

- Pair with a nude lipstick of choice.

When removing eye gems, use your fingers or tweezers and pop them back in their original packet so you can reuse them.

COLOURED SMOKY EYE

A classic smoky eye but with a twist! Instead of using neutral or black to create a smoky eye, switch things up and go for a colour. Think about what outfit you're wearing and what could work. I particularly love a jewelled purple, deep blue or emerald green. And to give it more of a party feel I love adding a shimmer onto the lid instead of keeping it matte. Let me show you how to create a blue sparkly smoky eye.

- Apply your base makeup and brows and prime the eye area.

- Blend a navy eyeshadow all over your lid, into your crease and upwards towards your brow. Take this shade as high as you want, but make sure you leave space below the brow. If you want even more depth, switch to using a black eyeshadow.

- Take this shade along the underneath of your lower lash line as well.

- Take a mid blue eyeshadow and pop it on your lid, diffusing into the navy/black in your crease.

- Then take a blue metallic or glitter liquid eyeshadow and pat that all over your lid for the sparkle.

- Take a kohl eyeliner in black and line your waterline for maximum impact.

- Apply mascara or false lashes to finish off the eyes.

- I find when you've gone bold and dramatic on your eyes, it's best to keep to a light nude lip.

This smoky eye technique works really well with any shade, as long as you're going darker on the crease and outer edge of the eye and lighter on the lid.

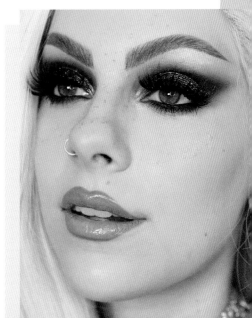

Daytime

Daytime makeup, depending on the occasion, can be slightly different to what you'd wear in the evening. You might opt for more neutrals, something glowy or even pastel. You might be attending a wedding as a guest, having a summer BBQ with friends and family or just a day out. Here are four makeup looks to get you inspired for all your daytime occasions.

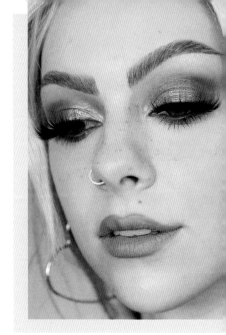

ROSE GOLD

Rose gold is a gorgeous colour for daytime makeup. It works well on all complexions and adds warmth and radiance to your skin. It's a beautiful tone to wear as a wedding guest and it's just enough colour if you're wanting something in between neutral and bright.

- Apply your base makeup with a pink blush, do your brows and prime your eye area.

- Apply a mid pink matte eyeshadow all over your lid, diffusing up to just below the brow. Bring that shadow down and underneath the eye.

- Apply a slightly deeper pinky nude hue to the crease, outer lid area and underneath your eye to add depth.

- Apply a rose gold metallic shimmer over your lid either with a powder or liquid eyeshadow.

- Add a pop of highlight to the inner corner of your eye.

- Add a dark brown kohl eyeliner to your waterline.

- Add a dark brown eyeshadow to along the top lash line.

- Add mascara or false lashes.

- Add a pinky nude lip to finish.

My top picks:
Affordable: Makeup Revolution Reloaded Provocative
Mid-range: Morphe 18V Va-Va Bloom Artistry Palette
High-end: Urban Decay Naked Cherry Palette
Sustainable: ROEN Beauty Eyeshadow Palette

GLOWY NEUTRAL

A neutral, glowy makeup look is always a great option for the day, especially when paired with a sweep of gold metallic eyeshadow across the lids. Wearing gold within your eye makeup will pair well with gold jewellery and warm up the skin.

- Apply your base makeup with bronzed cheeks and golden highlight, do your brows and prime your eye area.

- Sweep a mid to deep brown into your crease, diffusing up towards your brow bone, and wing it out.

- Take a metallic gold liquid eyeshadow and sweep it over your lid, diffusing into your crease.

- Optional – apply a black or brown winged liner from your inner corner and wing it out as much as you like.

- Buff a dark brown eyeshadow to add depth to the outer part of underneath your lash line.

- Add a dark brown or black kohl eyeliner to your waterline.

- Add mascara or false lashes.

- Add a nude lip with a golden sparkly gloss.

To add even more glow to this look, you could pick a setting spray with a gold shimmer.

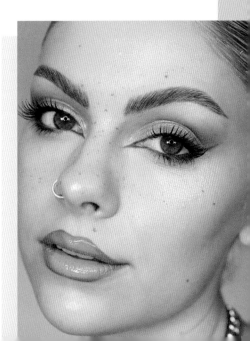

BRONZE EYE, RED LIP

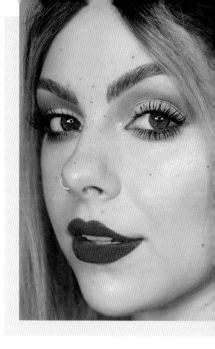

You don't always need to keep your eyes bare or opt for a winged liner when paired with a red lip. A bronzed, neutral eye can also complement a statement red lip and warm up your complexion.

- Apply your base makeup with bronzed cheeks and a golden highlight, do your brows and prime your eye area.

- Blend a mid to deep brown into your crease, diffusing up towards your brow bone. Keep the shadow around the outer eye rounded and bring it underneath your lower lashes.

- Sweep a light cream eyeshadow from the inner corner to the centre of your lid so it transitions into the deeper shadow.

- Add a golden pop of highlight into the inner corner.

- Apply mascara or false lashes.

- Apply a statement red lip. For a day look I tend to opt for a satin formula as it gives your lips a more natural finish.

A red lip can really elevate a neutral eye; it adds glam but keeps it super-wearable for the day.

SOFT GLAM

Soft glam is quite literally *soft*. No harsh lines, diffused eyeshadows, glowing skin, fluffy brows and neutral eyes. With a soft, glam makeup look, everything is blended seamlessly into the skin. It's perfect for a day occasion and suits all skin tones and eye colours.

- When applying your base makeup, opt for a sheer foundation and use concealer for the extra coverage in areas if you need to.

- With a large sponge gently add depth to just under the cheekbones using a bronzer a few shades deeper than your skin tone. Using a sponge will blend it into your skin without any harsh lines.

- Add a neutral blush to the apples of the cheeks and a golden highlight to the highest part of the cheekbone.

- Keep brows bushy, brush through brow gel and fill in any sparse areas creating hair-like strokes.

- To start off your eye look, prime the eye area.

- Start by buffing a matte deep neutral hue into the crease and upwards towards the brow, leaving space underneath.

- Buff concealer lightly over the lid and gently blend into the crease, in a curved shape.

- Take a light neutral matte eyeshadow and pat over the top of the concealer.

- Define your eye shape with a thin line of liquid eyeliner and wing out slightly.

- Add mascara or false lashes.

- Finish off with a nude lip, paired with a lip liner in a few shades deeper.

You want to keep everything neutral with a soft glam look with similar hues, so your lips match the tone of your cheeks and eyes.

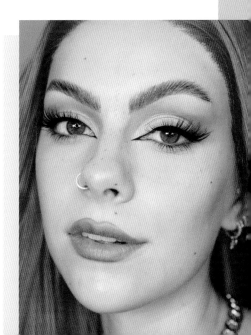

Holiday

When it comes to holiday makeup, I love to change it up every night. It's an opportunity to take your time getting ready, there's no rush of daily life. I've got a few makeup look ideas for your next holiday, whether you're partying it up and wanting something fun or you want that golden-hour glow.

NEON

Neon makeup is such a fun colour palette to wear on a summer holiday and it actually suits all skin tones. Neon eye makeup is bold and there are so many ways you can tie it into different looks

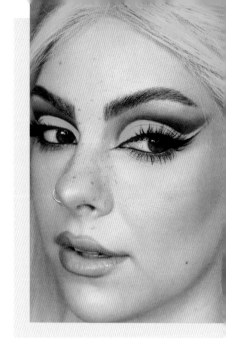

- Prime your skin, you want to make sure it's sweatproof!

- Apply your chosen base makeup and brows with bronzed cheeks and a golden highlight and prime your eye area.

- Apply a matte dark green eyeshadow just above your eye crease, wing it out and blend upwards towards your brow. Make sure to leave space below your brow.

- Use concealer to create a sharp, defined cut crease, winging it out.

- Pack on a neon green eyeshadow on your lid and up to where you've cut the crease.

- Apply a liquid eyeliner along the lash line, wing it out at the outer and inner eye.

- Apply a metallic green eyeshadow just below the inner eye wing and bring it back into the undereye.

- Apply mascara or false lashes and a nude glossy lip.

PEACHY

Peachy tones look incredible on every skin tone and go hand in hand with summer. They add softness to your look while giving a natural glow and are a great go-to for holiday makeup. If you're fair-skinned you might want to pick a peachy pastel hue and if you're dark go for deep corals. There are quite a few ways to incorporate this fruity shade into your makeup looks through blusher, eye makeup and lips – or combining all three. I love when your entire look is peach-themed so try this next time you're getting holiday ready.

- Prime your skin well to make sure your base is sweat- and humidity proof.

- Apply your chosen base makeup and brows.

- Sweep a peachy blush over the apples of your cheeks and pair with a golden glowy highlight on the cheekbones.

- Prime the eye area.

- Apply your chosen peachy matte eyeshadow all over your lid.

- Take a slightly deeper peachy shade and apply into your crease, blending upwards towards your brow.

- Apply an inner corner highlight with the highlighter you used on your cheekbones.

- Add mascara or false lashes.

- Apply a peachy nude lip with a clear gloss.

- A super-easy and flattering holiday makeup look that will leave you glowing and sun-kissed.

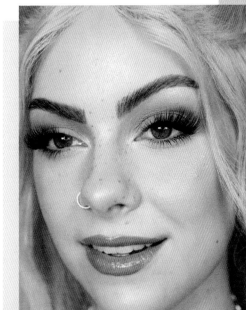

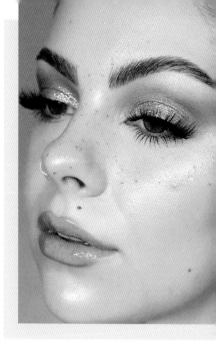

GOLDEN HOUR GLOW

Want even more of a glow? Switch up the peachy tones for gold. You know when the sun is setting and a magical golden glow illuminates everything? You can achieve just that with makeup. There's nothing more flattering than a golden complexion and a glowing highlight.

- Prime your skin well to make sure your base is sweat- and humidity proof.

- Apply your base makeup and, to really give your skin that golden glow, mix in an illuminator with your foundation before applying.

- Apply a sheer liquid bronzer and golden liquid highlighter to add depth and highlight.

- To lock makeup in place, opt for a setting powder that's lightweight and illuminating. Some have glitter or light-refracting pigments that add to the glow.

- Do your eyebrows and prime your eye area.

- Here's where we add even more gold into the look. Apply a matte deep neutral shadow into your crease and upwards towards your brow, leaving space underneath.

- Add depth into the crease with a dark brown to black shadow.

- Sweep a gold metallic eyeshadow over the eyelid. Apply gold glitter over the top.

- Add mascara or false lashes.

- Apply a chosen nude lip with a sparkly gold gloss.

- Finish off with a gold illuminating setting spray.

A glowy look, perfect for that golden hour. And if you want to add even more glow? Match your body to your face's glow by using a body luminiser cream or spray.

Festival

I'm known for many things in the online world and being a 'Festival Queen' is one of them. I love the freedom and creativity that a festival brings and a key part for me, is the makeup, hair and outfit.

On this occasion, anything goes – it's the perfect time to experiment! There have been festival makeup trends over the years, but in all honesty you can wear whatever you like, whether that's fancy dress, donning yourself head to toe in glitter or keeping things minimal. Everyone has their own festival style; it's a place where people from all different backgrounds come together for the music and I love seeing the looks everyone creates.

For me, I always like a theme, and first I'll see if the festival I'm attending has one – some do – for example, it might be 'Love', so I think about lots of references such as rainbow, hearts, reds/pink, Cupid. Or I pick my outfit first, then I let the fabric inspire me. It might have stars on it, be neon in colour or rainbow. I like everything matching and tied together, so once I have my theme, I start to plan my looks around it.

Here are some of my favourite festival themes.

RAINBOW

If you want a super-colourful theme, rainbow is a great choice. If you can't pick one colour, why not wear them all? A really bold and playful theme where you could create a rainbow eyeshadow or eyeliner look. Or even wear rainbow face jewels! There are so many different looks you could create with this theme in mind.

- Prime your skin well to make sure your base is sweatproof – you're going to be boogieing at a festival, so you want your makeup to last.

- Apply your chosen base makeup and brows.

- Apply a rainbow gradient of eyeshadow just above your cut crease, following the shape of your eye and winging it out. Start with red from the inner corner, blending into the rest of the rainbow shades, ending with purple.

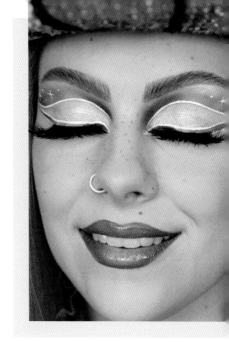

- Take your concealer and cut the edge of the crease, making sure it's sharp and defined.

- Apply a white shimmer eyeshadow over the top of the lid.

- Apply rainbow eyeliner in the same gradient as the crease, starting with red and working way along the rainbow, ending with purple.

- Repeat the rainbow gradient but apply under the eye and join the outer wing.

- Add white kohl eyeliner to the waterline.

- Add mascara or false lashes.

- Finish with a bold, matte red lipstick.

If you want to go even bolder you can add white stars around the eyes, glitter or gems, or even rainbow lashes!

BUTTERFLY

From dainty pastels to bold, colourful butterfly wing designs, you can really make this eye makeup your own. Whether you go dramatic with a sharp black outline or keep it soft with a white liner, once you've mastered drawing the shape of butterfly wings around your eyes, you can just keep experimenting.

- Prime your eye area.

- Use a brown kohl eyeliner pencil and lightly mark out your wing shape around your eyes.

- Once you're happy, go over it in a black liquid eyeliner.

- Now you can go in with eyeshadow on your lid. You could pick one colour or create a gradient with a few. Take the colour further than your eyelid and colour in the wings.

- Taking your black eyeliner again, you're going to start marking out the pattern within the wings. You want to create lines that join up and create circular shapes. Once you've got your wings marked out, you want to define the lines and thicken the edge of the wings.

- Line your lash line with black eyeliner.

- Apply different-sized white dots to the black edge of the wings.

- Apply a white, black or colour kohl eyeliner to your waterline.

- Apply mascara or false lashes.

- Finish with a lipstick that complements the look.

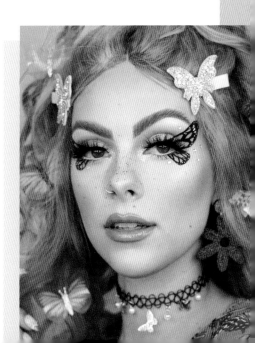

If you want to add to this you could glue down some rhinestones around the eyes or even outline the edge of the butterfly wing shape.

FLOWERS

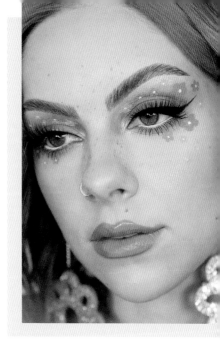

Flower eye makeup is really easy to create and looks super-cute. You can play around with different colour palettes and the positioning of the flowers.

- Prime your skin and create your chosen base makeup and brows with a blush shade that's going to complement your colour scheme. If you're going for orange flowers, for example, opt for a peachy blush.

- Prime the eye area. Pick one eyeshadow colour and apply it all over your lid, blending upwards towards your brow and underneath your eye.

- Apply a wing liner in your chosen style.

- Add a pop of highlight to the inner corner of your eye.

- To create the flowers, either grab a face or body paint palette or liquid eyeliner. I prefer using a face or body palette as I can use a thin, precise liner brush to paint the flowers on – sometimes the nibs of liquid eyeliners can be too thick. Choose one or a few colours for the petals and start painting on simple flower shapes randomly around the eye. A good tip here is mark out four or five dots that will make the petals, then join them together and colour them in.

- Once you've applied the main flower shape, take white or other colours of choice and draw a dot in the centre of each shape.

- Apply mascara or false lashes and a lipstick of choice to complement the look – either use a colour within the same shades as the eye look or go for a nude to keep the focus on the eyes.

This makeup really gives off a retro 60s feel. If you want something a little more subtle, try drawing small flowers along the top of your lash line and winging it out – flower eyeliner! Or keep your eyes simple and draw one small daisy flower with white and yellow underneath the centre of both eyes.

OG *EUPHORIA* LOOK

When the HBO hit TV show *Euphoria* reached our screens it spiralled into viral *Euphoria*-themed makeup looks being recreated all over social media – think glitter pigments, rhinestone embellishments, sharp graphic liner looks.

- Prime your skin and create your chosen base makeup and brows. For that extra *Euphoria* glow, add a glittery highlight to the high points of your face.

- Prime your eye area.

- Create a cut crease of your colour choice, pick three shades of the same hue – light, mid and deep. Start by applying your deepest eyeshadow along the edge of where you want the cut crease to start. Follow your eye shape and wing it out towards the tail end of your brow. Use a small blending brush to blend up towards your brow. Take this colour under your eye.

- Cut your crease with concealer, keep it sharp and wing it out. Apply your lightest eyeshadow colour over the top of the concealer.

- Take a few different-sized rhinestones in your colour choice. Use eyelash glue to adhere and a wax gem applicator to easily pick up the rhinestones. Apply them along where you created your cut crease. Start with smaller rhinestones on the inner eye, and as you work your way along in slightly larger rhinestones. Once you reach the end of the wing, take the rhinestones back in towards the eye.

- Apply eyeliner along your top lash line and take it out past the inner corner of the eye. Add kohl eyeliner to the waterline, then mascara or false lashes.

- Finish with a nude lipstick and add a glitter gloss for that extra sparkle.

The addition of rhinestones within a makeup look really does elevate it. You'll definitely catch people's eyes with this look.

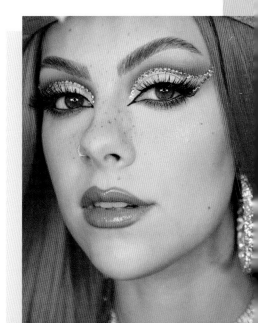

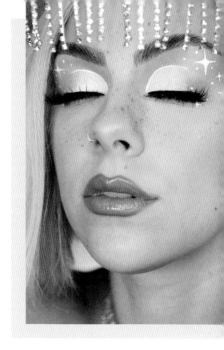

PASTEL

Dreamy pastels are mesmerising for a festival. Think pastel clouds, stars, fairies or even a pastel rainbow.

I particularly love pastel pink, blue and lilac together, so here's a dreamy eye makeup look to try out.

- Prime your skin and create your chosen base makeup and brows with a colour for blush that's going to complement your chosen colour scheme. With these particular pastels a pink blush works well.

- Prime the eye area.

- Apply a pastel pink into blue into lilac eyeshadow gradient in your crease and blend upwards towards the brow. Start from the inner eye and take it out towards the tail end of the brow.

- Apply a concealer and create a half cut crease. Make the cut defined up to just over halfway across the eye's crease.

- Pack a white eyeshadow on top of where you applied concealer and blend out towards the end of the eye. Then take the lilac eyeshadow and pack it into the white to seamlessly transition the colours at the end of the eyelid. Add a glitter pigment on top of this white shadow for a sparkle.

- Blend the same pink, blue and lilac gradient under the eye.

- Add a white kohl eyeliner into the waterline.

- Add a white liquid liner along the edge of the cut crease.

- Draw a few white stars and dots on the outer of the eye.

- Line the top lash line with a black liquid liner.

- Add mascara or false lashes.

- Choose either a pastel lipstick to match the eyeshadow colours or a nude.

FESTIVAL MAKEUP HACKS

Face gems won't stick? Glitter all over your face at the end of the night? Felt like a sweaty mess while dancing? I've got some great hacks for you that will help your festival makeup last all day long and avoid you seeing the remnants of yesterday's look the next day.

HACK 1 – WATERPROOF MAKEUP

You can't predict the weather, and if it rains, you won't want your makeup to run. Opt for waterproof eyeliner and mascara and take it even further by applying a waterproof foundation/concealer. If you're prepared, you'll still look glam in the rain.

HACK 2 – TAKING OFF YOUR GLITTER

Before you grab your makeup remover and wipe that glitter – STOP! When packing your makeup bag for your festival weekend, always remember some sticky tape, which you can use to remove your glitter before going in with your makeup remover. That way you won't smear it all over your face and be covered in it all weekend. I mean, that's what most of us want at festivals, but glitter can get EVERYWHERE, and you don't want to be bringing it home with you – trust me!

HACK 3 – MINIS!

If you're doing a three-day festival and camping, take travel-sized beauty products or even testers with you. And if you don't have any of those, collect small refillable containers throughout the year so you can decant your products into them at no extra cost. You don't want to weigh your bag down with heavy makeup that you've got to lug halfway across a field.

HACK 4 – MULTI-FUNCTIONAL PRODUCTS

When packing for a festival, try to think about one product that can do a lot of things. For example, got2b hair gel is a great product because you can use it for your brows, hairstyles and even as a glue for glitter.

Halloween

Another time of year when we can experiment and get creative with makeup, where anything goes! You have the freedom to turn yourself into any character you choose and you can have fun with it. I've always loved Halloween. Fancy dress for me is so exciting, and I plan my looks months in advance and count down the days until I can get into my costume.

Halloween can be daunting for some, though. Who are you going to be? And how are you going to create the look? I find that as long as you've got Halloween makeup on in some capacity, the rest of your outfit doesn't matter too much, and it will all come together.

Halloween makeup doesn't need to involve special effects and liquid latex. If you're skilled with using those types of products – amazing! You can create some scary looks with them. If you're just wanting to master an easy but effective Halloween look, though, I've got you sorted! And you won't need to run to the store for any extra beauty supplies – you can just use the makeup you've already got. If you want to elevate your simple looks, invest in coloured or patterned contact lenses. Applying red, white and black contacts to a Halloween look instantly adds a sense of spookiness. And if you're wanting to really get creative, I highly recommend buying a face and body paint oil palette like the one from UCANBE Athena.

HALLOWEEN MAKEUP HACKS

Before I get into sharing some Halloween makeup ideas with you, let's start with the basics. These hacks might take a little practice to nail, but once you've got them down to a T, you will be able to apply them to so many different looks in the future.

HACK 1 – BLOCKING OUT YOUR BROWS

Creating a Halloween look that's going to cover your brows? Or maybe you're turning yourself into a character whose eyebrows are a different shape to yours. Learning how to block out your brows is a really helpful technique.

- Make sure your skin is bare and your brows are free of product.

- Brush your brow hairs up and completely cover them with glue. The purple disappearing glue from Elmer's is great. Make sure you keep brushing up your

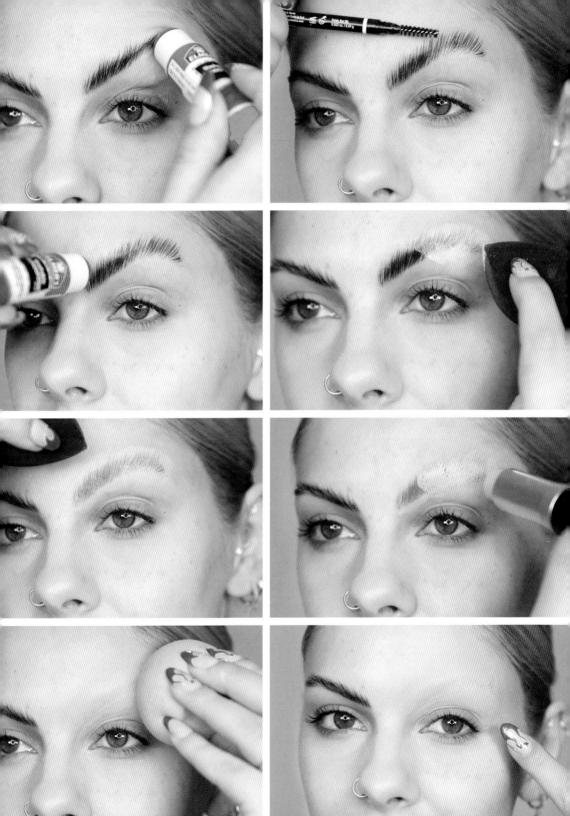

brow hairs while applying the glue so they are lying flat against your skin. Apply a few coats of adhesive.

- Taking a loose setting powder, you want to press the powder into the glued brows using a sponge. Press it on over the whole eyebrow until it's completely covered in powder. Dust off any excess with a fluffy makeup brush.

- If you're keeping your skin to your natural tone and wearing foundation, apply a stick foundation over the top of the glue/powdered brows to conceal them. Make sure you swipe in the direction of how you've laid your brow hairs. Use a setting powder to set.

- If you're not keeping your skin tone natural and are maybe painting yourself white for a skull look or red for a devil, you can go straight in with your face/body paint after you've covered your glued brows with setting powder.

And that's how easy it is! The key to blocking out your brows is to make sure your hairs are flat against your skin and the glue is applied smoothly so you cannot see any hairs and it looks flat once concealed.

HACK 2 – APPLYING SILICONE PROSTHETICS

If you're wanting to go down the special FX route with your Halloween makeup, try silicone prosthetics. They're on the slightly more expensive scale of prosthetic, but they look really realistic and are a lot easier to apply. Types of silicone prosthetic you might find online are devil horns, mermaid scales or gills, rotting flesh or even noses.

Silicone is a lightweight material, flexible and translucent. The edges of silicone can be easily blended into the skin. The only downside is you tend to not be able to get more than one use out of them, but then how often are you going to be doing special FX makeup?

- Decide where you'll be applying the prosthetic then clean and dry the area thoroughly.

- Gently remove your silicone prosthetic from the packaging and flip it over.

- Apply a thin layer of silicone adhesive to the contact side of the prosthetic, right out to the edge. They key here is to not apply too much.

- Apply a thin layer to your skin where you're going to place the prosthetic.

- Allow plenty of time for the adhesive to dry – this is the key to it staying put. Once dry to the touch, apply the prosthetic to the skin. Try to keep the thin edges up and press down from the centre. You want to make sure there are no bubbles and all the air is removed. Start in the centre and work your way out to the edges. Once applied smoothly, press down firmly.

- Take some acetone to blend out the edges. Silicone prosthetics will come with a thick edge of silicone around the design, the acetone will dissolve this off. Take a cotton bud for this step and dip one end in acetone. Wipe this onto the edge of the silicone all around the outside and it'll melt and blend into the skin. Acetone is very drying to the skin so try to avoid getting it on your own skin if you can.

- Once the prosthetic edges are blended, apply a loose setting powder around the edges to remove any leftover tackiness.

- Then go in with your foundation, face paint, fake blood – whatever you need to finish off your desired look.

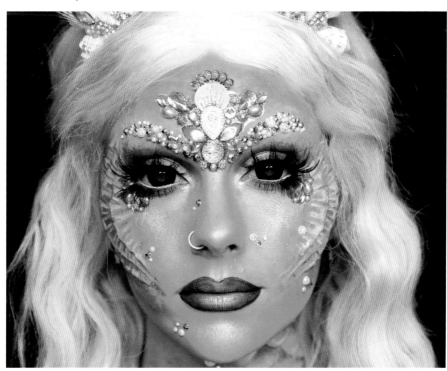

HACK 3 – FAKE BLOOD

Fake blood is a lot of people's go-to for a Halloween look. It can look really effective applied in different ways and I have a few tricks for you to try. Either DIY your own blood by mixing together red lipstick of your choice, a creamy black kohl eyeliner and clear lip gloss – start off with the red lipstick and add small amounts of black eyeliner to your desired blood shade before adding the gloss – or grab some fake blood from your local fancy dress shop. The fake blood I find most realistic is a coagulated blood gel, as it doesn't stain your skin and is a thick gel-like formula that really resembles realistic blood.

The first way I like to add blood is by applying a thick dot onto a fake wound, from my eyes or sides of my lips. Because it's a thick dot, it will trickle – let it do this naturally so it looks realistic, rather than brushing it on.

Another technique that works well is creating a blood splatter. You will want a watery blood formula for this – red face paint works well. Take two makeup brushes, one with the product on and another that you will use to push back the bristles on the brush with the product on, so you can flick it back at your face, creating that blood splatter effect. Super-easy and effective.

HACK 4 – LIQUID LATEX

Liquid latex is a versatile product when it comes to special FX and Halloween makeup. You can do a lot with it, however it can be challenging to work with. It comes in a variety of shades to resemble skin tones but also comes in other colours, such as white. It can be used for many things. You want to add a wound on your cheek? Maybe even a bullet hole in the centre of your forehead? I'm going to share a great tip on using liquid latex to create simple wounds, as these can add instant gore to your Halloween looks.

- Start with clean, dry skin and use a cotton bud to paint liquid latex onto your skin in the shape you want the wound to be.

- While the liquid latex is drying, rip up small pieces of tissue – you can use standard toilet roll – then lay these flat on top of the liquid latex, leaving a gap in the centre where the open wound will be. Then apply another layer of liquid latex over the top of the tissue.

- Let this dry – you can use a hairdryer to speed up the drying process; just remember not to have the heat set up too high, as you don't want to burn your face.

- Once dry, repeat steps 2 and 3 a few times. You want to build up the layers of latex and tissue, making sure the edges of the tissue are flat to the skin.

- Once completely dry, apply a setting powder over the top to remove any tackiness and shine.

- Tear into the latex in the centre to open up the wound shape.

- Apply foundation over the top of the tissue and latex to blend in with your skin colour.

- Apply different shades of eyeshadow inside the open part of the wound. Colours like dark purple/grey/reds work well.

- Add fake blood inside the open part of the wound and dripping from it. Now you've got a gory wound perfect for Halloween!

If you're allergic to latex, you could use a glue stick to create a small wound instead. Cut off a section of glue stick, mix with a little with water to mould it into a shape, then adhere it to your skin. Make sure you mark a hole in the centre of your shape for the eyeshadow and blood to go; you could even add some bruising around the edge with black/purple eyeshadow.

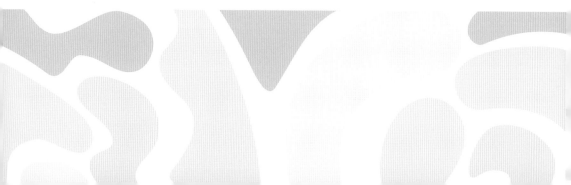

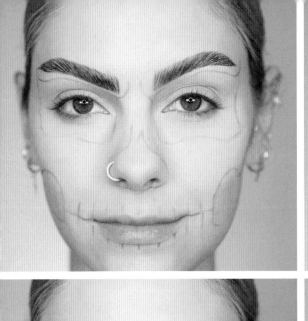
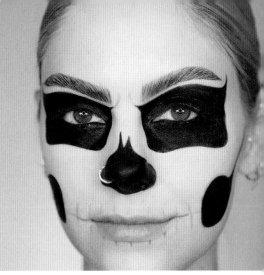
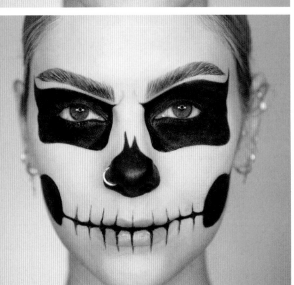
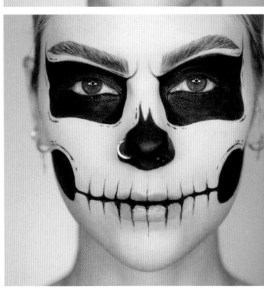
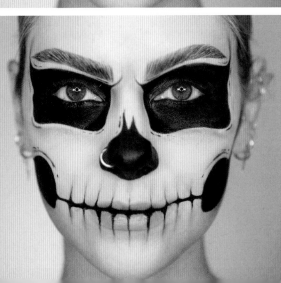
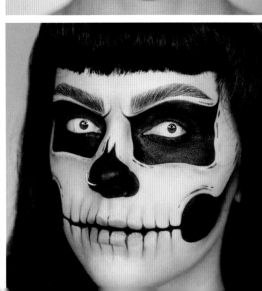

SKULL

Probably one of the most popular Halloween costumes is a skull. What I love most about this theme is the amount of ways you can work this into your look. You could go for a classic white/black skull, or do half glam/half skull or even a neon skull. Once you've mastered the technique, you can experiment and get creative.

Check out the easy, step-by-step guide opposite to help you master skull makeup and give you inspiration on how you can elevate your skull look to the next level.

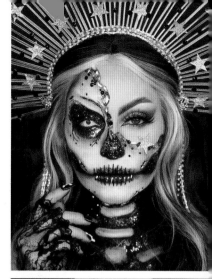

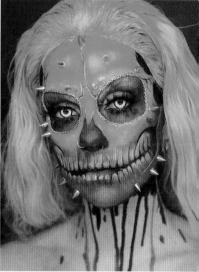

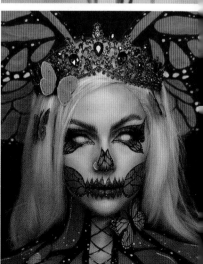

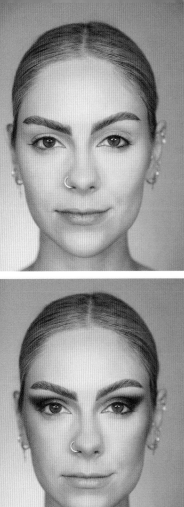
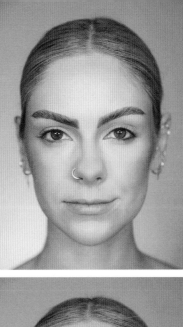
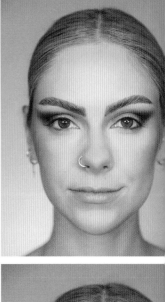
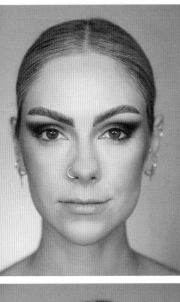
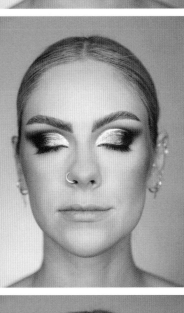
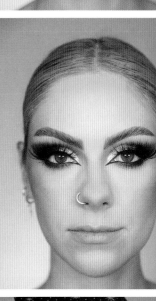
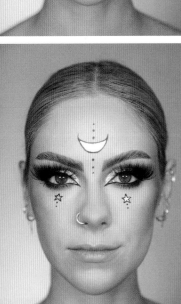
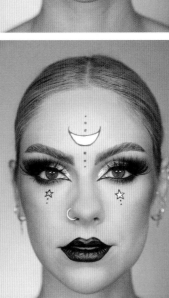
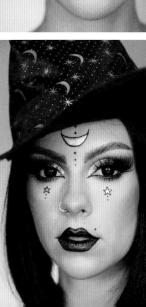

WITCH

Another popular costume choice for Halloween is a witch, and again, there are so many ways you could interpret this idea. You could go full-on *Hocus Pocus* or the Witch from *The Wizard of Oz*, or maybe be a glam, a goth or a mystical witch.

Here's a step-by-step of a spooky, mystical witch that's easy to recreate, and some more inspiration on other ways you can give yourself a witchy makeover.

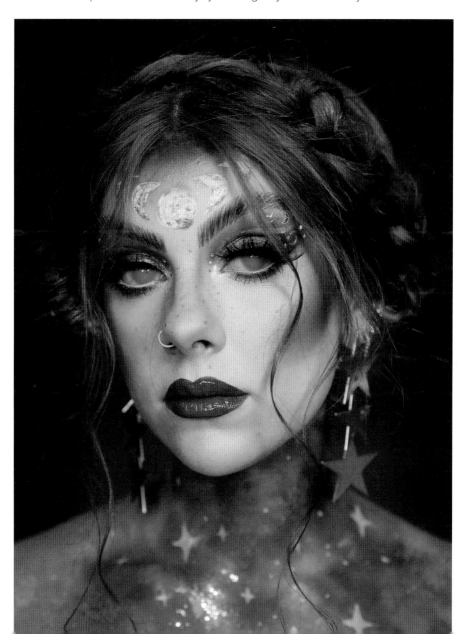

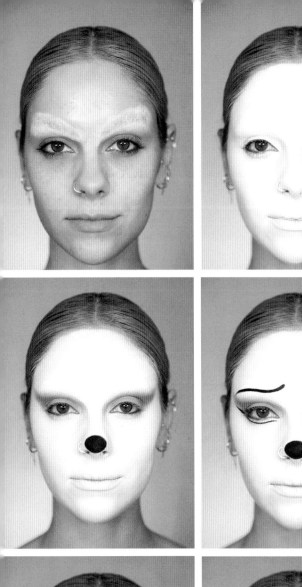
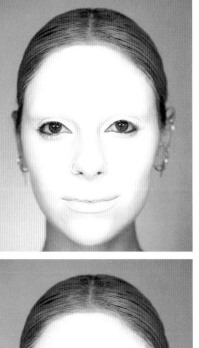
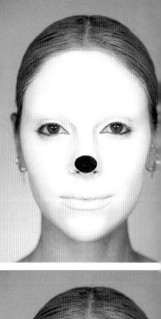
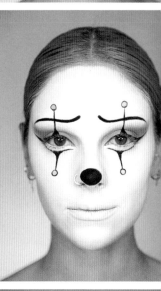
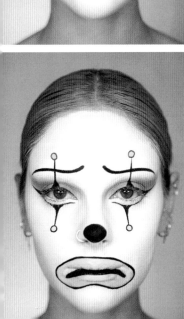
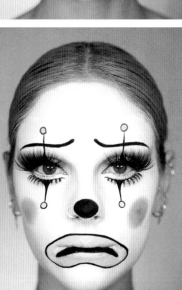
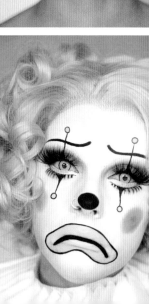

CLOWN

If clowns are your fear, then I'm sorry for what
you're about to see. Clowns are another great
costume idea for Halloween – let's be honest,
they're creepy and if you add blood and gore
they can be oh so terrifying.

Like every Halloween look, you can do your
own take on a clown. You could take inspiration
from films such as *IT* or from pantomimes or
create a Pierrot clown. My particular favourite
is a pastel sad clown, which I've given you a
super-easy step-by-step for. And if that doesn't
catch your eye, here's some more inspiration on
other ways to create a clown Halloween look.

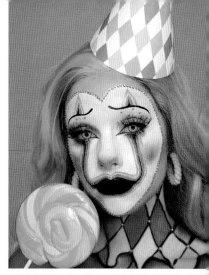

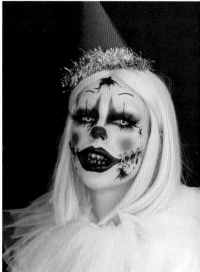

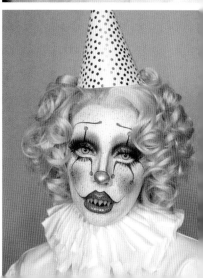

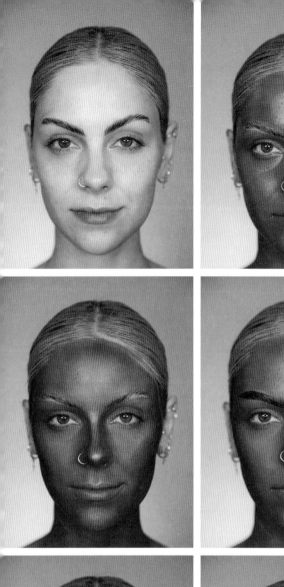
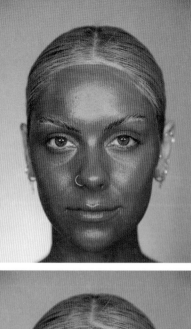
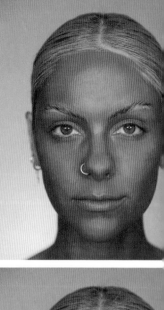
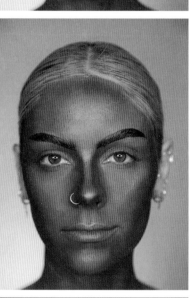
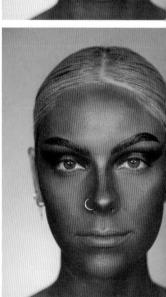
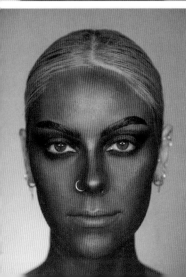
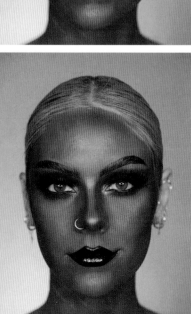
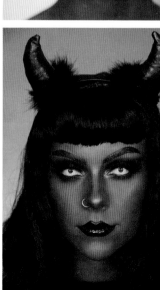

DEVIL

Lastly, we have this Halloween classic – a devil! You could let your outfit be the main part of your look and simply pair it with blood dripping from your eyes and red lips. Or you could go full-on devil glam. You can really turn a devil look into your own no matter what your makeup skill level or creativity.

Personally, my go-to for a Halloween devil is glam and painting myself red! It looks like a lot to do but with Athena face and body paint palette, it's super-easy. The oil paint essentially acts as your foundation/concealer so you can create a great red base and use a translucent setting powder to lock it in place. Then you devil glam it up.

Here's an easy-to-follow step-by-step for a devil glam look, plus some more inspiration if you fancy trying something else.

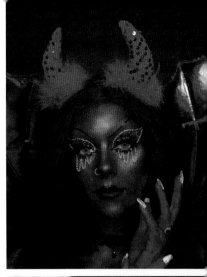

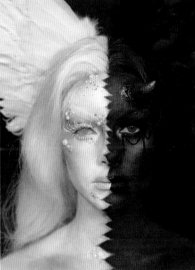

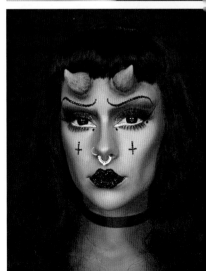

REMOVING HALLOWEEN MAKEUP

You'll use a lot of makeup to create some of your Halloween looks, especially if you're covering your face in paints, liquid latex and special FX. Removing it properly is key, so you're not putting your skin under stress.

I highly recommend investing in a good makeup and adhesive remover, the Ben Nye Remove-It All is great as it's universal and removes everything from cream makeups to spirit gum and prosthetic adhesives. It can be really enticing to just want to rip the prosthetic off your face, but please think about your skin!

With any prosthetics the best way to remove them is by using a cotton bud and remover and working around the edges to gently lift them away from the skin first. Once the edges are lifted, work the remover under the rest of the prosthetic, using your fingers in a circular motion, working it into your skin while lifting the prosthetic off. It will take a while, but it's a really beneficial step for your skin.

When removing liquid latex and tissue wounds, you don't necessarily need a dedicated remover for this, an oil-based makeup remover works well. Do the same technique as above and lift the edges first, then get your cotton bud right underneath the wound to lift it off. You'll probably find some remnant bits of liquid latex on your skin, so use a reusable makeup pad with remover on in a circular motion to break down the latex.

Once all your adhesive products are removed, you can then go in with a reusable makeup pad and makeup remover to remove the rest.

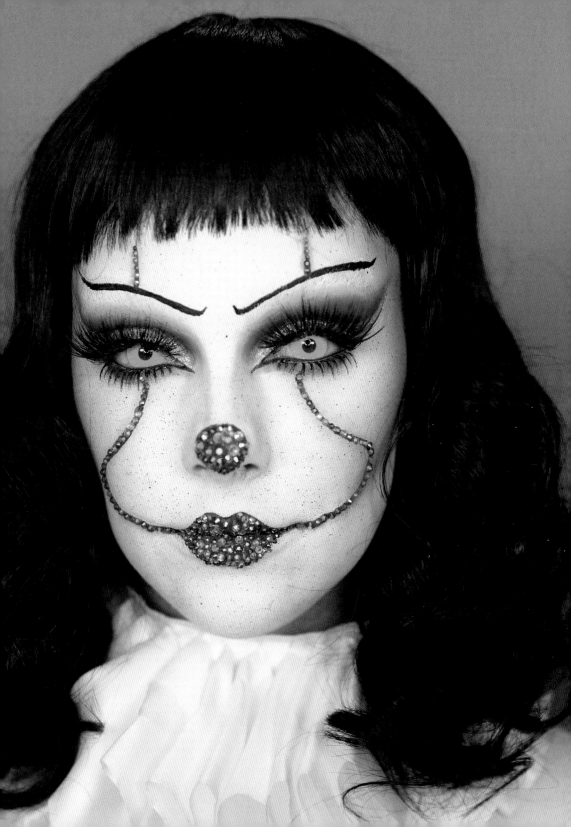

Inspiration

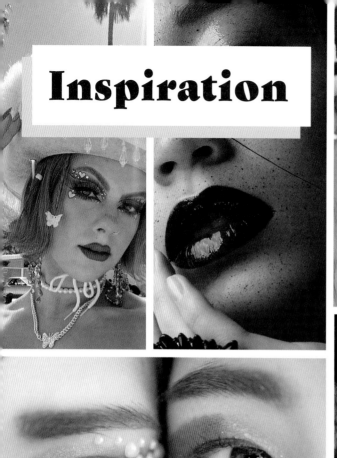
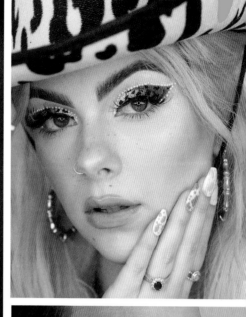
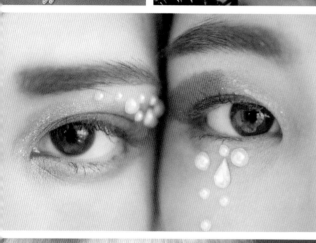
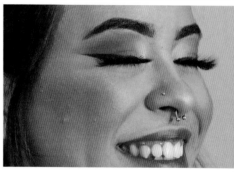
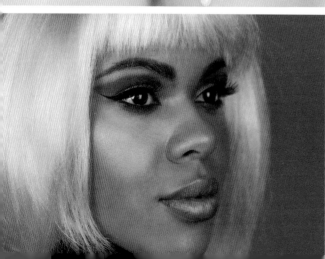
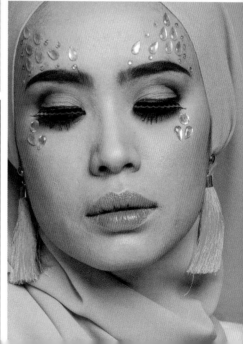

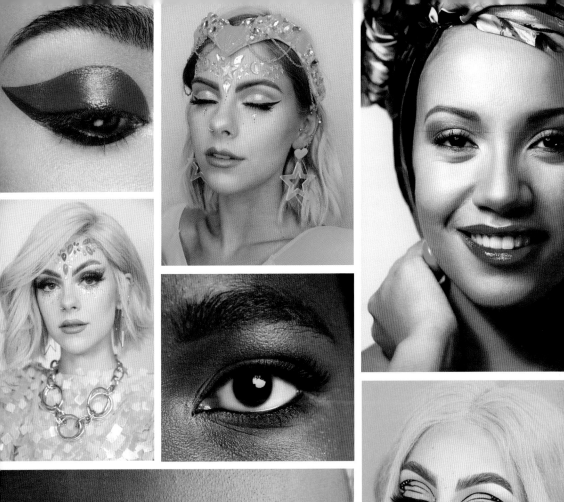
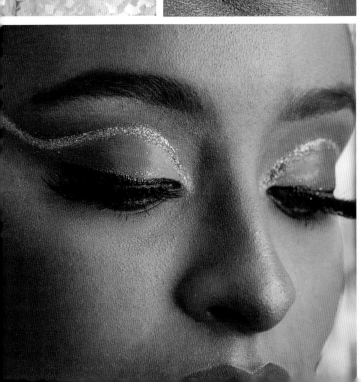
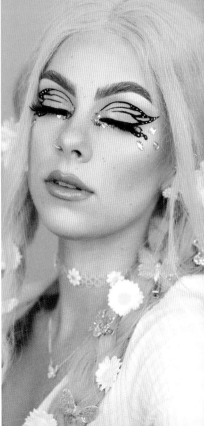

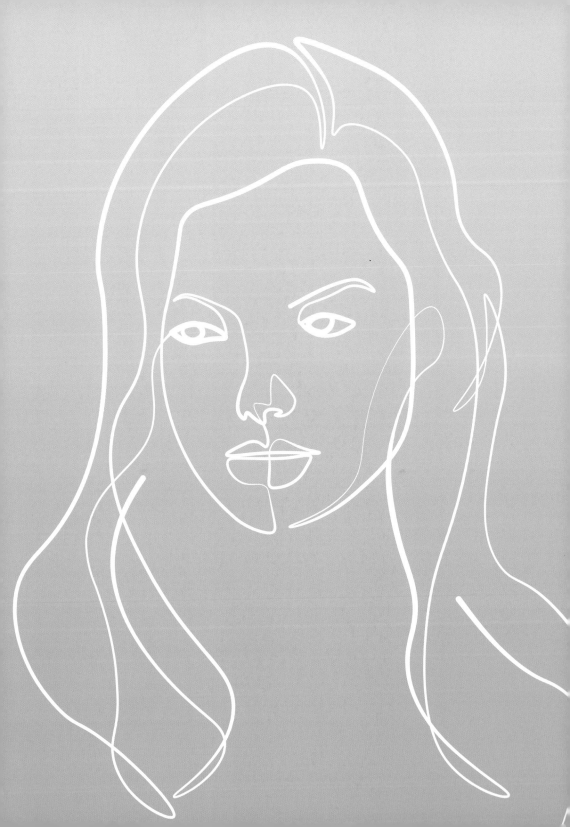

hair

Hair Kit

So you want to experiment with your hair? Maybe you want try out some new hairstyles. I've got some key tools that you're going to need before getting started. These are products I've found to be useful to have on hand from my 15-plus years of trying out different hairstyles and changing up my colour. Some might be more relevant to you than others, depending on your hair type and length, but you don't need to rush out the door and take this list straight to a shop. Your hair kit, like your makeup kit, can be built up over time.

STYLING PRODUCTS

If you're not using any styling products in your haircare routine, you might need to change things up. Styling products can offer protection against things like damage, heat and UV rays, which in turn improve the overall health of your hair. And not only this, styling products can help us achieve slick hairstyles, defined curls, volume, shine and just generally make our hair look fabulous.

This list is long… But I'm going to take you through some key beneficial hair styling products and why they're great for your hair. Now you won't need every single one of these – many offer a multitude of benefits in one, such as heat protection, shine, anti-frizz, strength and repair. I use a mix of high-street and high-end products – sometimes the more affordable option does exactly what you need it to do!

HEAT-PROTECT SPRAY

A heat-protecting spray is so important to use if you're using hairdryers, curlers or straighteners. A product like this will help minimise damage by adding a protective barrier. You can use it on wet or dry hair and most of these sprays offer other benefits like reducing split ends and adding shine. If your hair is bleached like mine, you will never want to miss this step; you need to avoid any further damage to your hair. A personal favourite is the VO5 Heat Protect Spray, it's affordable and comes in a large spray bottle that lasts me a while.

LEAVE-IN CONDITIONER OR TREATMENT

A leave-in conditioner is literally a conditioner you leave in, there's no rinsing it out. You apply it to towel-dried hair through a spray or cream and comb it through, and it can have amazing benefits. Look for one that's specific for your hair needs: dry, damaged, curly, fine, frizzy, bleached. There are so many on the market to choose from. I apply a leave-in conditioner or treatment once I get out the shower, around once a week, and I usually opt for either the Briogeo Don't Despair, Repair! Strength + Moisture leave-in Spray Hair Mask or the OUAI Leave-In Conditioner. A leave-in provides extra benefits that stay in the hair, offering protection from heat, adding moisture, as well as repairing, detangling and smoothing.

HAIR OIL

Another leave-in product that has amazing benefits is hair oil. Often the natural sebum our hair produces isn't enough to keep it hydrated because we put our hair through a lot with styling and dyeing. This is where a hair oil can be used to inject moisture and provide protection. As with any hair product, you need to pick an oil specific to your hair's needs, as not all benefit everyone. I'll take you through how to know what your hair needs later in the book. The most common hair oils are coconut, argan, jojoba, grapeseed, almond, avocado and olive. But there are many other ones with incredible benefits that you can either add to damp or dry hair. Applying oil to damp hair is the most effective as our hair is more absorbent when wet. However, if you find your dry hair looks frizzy or damaged, adding a hair oil here can smooth and add shine. Most people have a combination of hair issues, so experimenting with different oils and hair treatments is the key to finding one that works best for you.

Best oils for hair types:
Dry, dull hair: coconut, argan, jojoba, almond, olive, grapeseed
Dry scalp: jojoba, lavender, lemongrass
Damaged hair: coconut, jojoba, almond, olive
Hair loss: almond, grapeseed, lemongrass
Dandruff-prone hair: jojoba, almond, olive, grapeseed, lemongrass
Slow-growing hair: coconut, almond

With my bleached hair, I opt for a mix between coconut oil and argan oil and I love the OGX hair oils: Damage Remedy + Coconut Miracle Oil and Renewing+ Argan Oil of Morocco Penetrating Oil. They're affordable and leave my hair shiny, smooth and non-greasy.

Briana Campbell, an influencer with multi-textured curly hair, says 'adding certain oils to my scalp can help strengthen and speed up the growth of my hair. Some examples are Tea Tree Oil for dry scalp, Jamaican Castor Oil for split-end reduction, thicker hair and added moisture, Coconut Oil for softness and frizz reduction'.

SERUMS

A hair serum is a bit different to an oil. It's still a leave-in product but its focus is adding a protective layer to your hair that will smooth, add shine and protect against pollution. It's great at hiding split ends if you're yet to visit your hairdresser! When applying a serum it's usually applied on towel-dried hair, however there are some that can be applied to dry hair. Apply a few drops to your palms, rub together and smooth the hair down from roots to tips, combing afterwards to evenly distribute. You won't need to apply a serum daily, as it can cause greasiness. Keep your serums to wash days or if you have extremely unmanageable frizzy hair.

When incorporating a hair serum into my own routine, I look to sustainable haircare brand Davines. In particular, I use their MINU Hair Serum that's specific for coloured hair; it's moisturising and offers protection to keep coloured hair brighter for longer.

CREAMS

A hair cream can offer a variety of different benefits, such as curl-defining, smoothing, hydrating, adding shine, volume and heat protection, and give the hair a light hold. You want to find a cream that's specific to your hair's needs as there are so many to choose from. For example, a curl-defining cream is great for holding natural curls where you want that touchable look and feel. Some hair creams should be applied to damp hair, especially if you are using it for curls.

There are creams for dry hair, too, which tend to focus on 'finishing' your hair looks by smoothing and adding shine, but also have an array of nourishing benefits. I opt for a finishing cream if I've styled my hair straight, to make it look shiny and sleek.

'I add a curl cream/definer from root to tip, aim my head down and flip my hair over my face, then scrunch my curls upwards with my hands. From there, I just let it air dry and I'm done with the leave-out. The Miss Jessie's Multicultural Curls is my go-to curl cream; it works best when applied to hair that is still wet or damp. It's like a really smooth custard and my hair feels lightweight, soft and bouncy when fully it's in. Smells good too! And another favourite is the Bounce Curls Defining Butta: Extra Moisture. It defines my curls the absolute best by far. When first applied, it feels like it's not doing anything until it gets absorbed into my hair, then it does an amazing job making my individual curls look phenomenally defined and shiny and it lasts all day as well!'
**BRIANA CAMPBELL
(INFLUENCER)**

SCALP PRODUCTS

It's just as important to treat your scalp as it is your actual hair. Our scalps can become itchy, inflamed, shed white flakes or even feel dry. We shouldn't neglect them. There are many products that offer an array of benefits, targeting scalp skin concerns, thinning hair, product build-up or even promote hair growth.

I suffer with a dry scalp on occasions, especially after a bleach hair appointment. To target this I use Christophe Robin Cleansing Purifying Scrub around twice a month on wet hair, before I shampoo – it's formulated with sea salt, which is a natural exfoliant that removes impurities and restores the scalp's balance. It also helps with product build-up, which I get from time to time through styling my hair and using other scalp products such as a Grow Gorgeous Daily Growth Serum (which promotes hair growth) and Davines Energizing Thickening Tonic (which increases hair diameter, leaving hair looking fuller). I apply both of these scalp products before I start styling, either while my hair is damp after a hair wash, or while my hair is dry, in between hair-wash days.

Another scalp product I highly recommend is a scalp massager. Using one of these offers amazing benefits for your scalp – from stimulating hair growth to exfoliating and loosening dandruff. The more you can give your scalp a massage, the better. I like to use a scalp massager while I'm shampooing, as it helps keep the shampoo concentrated on my scalp and roots.

DETANGLING SPRAY

Looking for knot-free hair that's painless when you brush? Detangling sprays not only help you untangle your hair, they also have other amazing benefits such as reducing breakage and frizz and offering heat protection. They essentially coat your hair in moisture, which allows your brush to glide through, so a detangling spray is certainly going to leave your hair feeling smooth.

HAIRSPRAY

Hairspray has become a staple styling product over the years. From taming flyaways, to locking in your updos and curls, hairspray will keep your hairstyle intact all day long. It's a finishing product, so you use it as one of the last steps in your routine, and not only does it offer hold, hairspray can also add volume and protect your hair from humidity. Choosing a hairspray will depend on the overall finish and style you're wanting to achieve, for example flexible hold, freeze hold, lift, texture, anti-humidity or shine.

My top picks:
Flexible Hairspray: Colour Wow Cult Favorite Firm + Flexible Hairspray
For Curls: ghd Curly Ever After Curl Hold Spray
Extreme Hold: Schwarzkopf got2b Glued Blasting Freeze Spray

For a hold, there are a few tips and tricks to using hairspray. If you're curling your hair, you might want to spray after each individual curl, and for flyaways you might want to spray a toothbrush (a clean one, of course) with hairspray, then brush the hairs down. If you want volume, tip your head upside down before spraying.

The key with hairspray is to avoid spraying too close to your hair. The best way to use it is to hold it around 15–20cm away and mist it over the area you're styling or where you want the hold.

If you do want hold and are looking for a more natural finish on the hair, you might want to try texture or beach spray. These can be used on damp or dry hair and give your hair that 'outta the sea' look without drying out your locks.

DRY SHAMPOO

For those days where you just don't fancy going through the process of washing and drying your hair, or maybe you've worked up a sweat in the gym, dry shampoo is a saviour. It can give your hair a refresh between wash days or if you want to extend the life of a blow-dry you've just had done. Dry shampoo is formulated with alcohol or starch and essentially soaks up the oils and grease in your hair, giving it a new lease of life and an extra day before you need to wash it again. Dry shampoo isn't meant to 'clean' your hair like a normal shampoo, so make sure you're not using it as a replacement for washing your hair. It's ok to use dry shampoo once or twice a week though. When using it, shake the can before spraying onto your sectioned roots and hold it about 15–20cm away from your hair. Once you've sprayed your roots, massage in the product using your fingers. Try to avoid using dry shampoo on multiple days in a row, as it can lead to product build-up and clog the pores on your scalp.

My top brands:
Affordable: *Colab*
Organic: *FeGoo*
Eco-Conscious: *Foamie*

You can find dry shampoo in many forms, the most obvious is as a spray, but if you're wanting to be more environmentally conscious, there are some great powders that come in cardboard shaker-style packaging or are formulated using organic ingredients.

MOUSSE

This is a foam product that is bouncy and light. It's used to give the hair some hold, add volume and definition, as well as protect and tame. When using a mousse you want to add a small ball of the formula to towel-dried hair from root to tip. If I want to create a voluminous, bouncy, blow-dry look, mousse is a great styling product. If you've got curly hair, use a diffuser on your hairdryer, and if you've got straight hair, use a rounded brush and you'll be able to create volume at the root by gently pulling the hair upwards while drying it.

When it comes to choosing a mousse, you can honestly achieve the look you want with the cheapest product. A higher price point tends to just mean more ingredients. Boots' own range of mousse is so affordable and does exactly what each one says on the bottle, and the bonus is that it doesn't leave your hair crunchy or with a sticky residue.

GELS AND WAX

A hair gel will help to set your hair in a specific style, lock it in place and prevent flyaways. You could use hairspray, but gel is great at providing long-lasting hold. You use gel a bit differently to hairspray as you apply it to damp hair and when your hair dries, the gel dries. Your hair is more manageable when it's damp; however, be careful if your hair is bleached as it tends to be extra vulnerable when wet. Make sure you use a water-soluble formula as it's easier to wash out. I use hair gel if I'm trying to achieve a wet-look finish or create an updo. Using gel is great for hair that's short, has bangs or layers that don't quite make it into a ponytail and need taming and locking into place.

Hair wax is a styling product that will keep your hair in place. You can achieve a strong hold but without the firm-hair-gel feel. Using a wax before braiding is a great hack as it gives your hair grip and makes it easier to style. It's also good for taming flyaways. When using a hair wax, you only need a small pea-sized amount. Rub it between your hands to warm the wax, then brush the surface of your hair to coat it. Then you can pat down flyaways, braid or run your fingers through to slick your hair into your desired style.

UV PROTECTION SPRAY

You protect your skin from harsh UV rays, so why wouldn't you protect your hair? The sun can cause a lot of damage to your hair, which can lead to breakage and contributes to colour fading. All hair types can experience damage, no matter the colour or texture. But if your hair is fine or light-coloured like mine, it's even more vulnerable as it's more fragile and prone to sun damage. Too much sun exposure can lead to the hair cuticle being damaged and also the breakdown of keratin, which is a natural protein in your hair – which bleach already strips from it.

To protect from sun and heat exposure, either wear a hat or hair scarf or use a UV protection spray. They're usually lightweight mists that form a protection barrier on the hair to minimise damage and dryness and that you apply to dry hair.

BRUSHES AND COMBS

Let's talk brushes and combs – both are great for detangling and styling. The trick is picking the right one for your needs and what you want to achieve.

COMBS

All-purpose comb – a handy comb that's split down the centre. One side has wider teeth and on the other the teeth are closer together. You can use it for detangling and quick combing but also finishing off hairstyles.

Wide-tooth comb – teeth are far apart. It's great for gently combing masks and conditioners or styling products through the hair and also detangling and combing through curls.

Fine-tooth comb – teeth are very close together. It's great for styling and pulling hair into place.

Detangler comb – a wide-tooth comb but with two rows of teeth to detangle quickly.

Pick comb – shaped like a painter's brush, it's a comb used for curly, thick or textured hair.

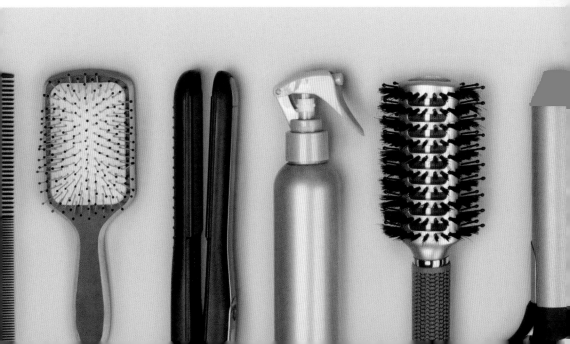

Rake comb – designed for thick, curly, frizzy hair. It's great for detangling but keeping curls in shape. It's adopted its name because of the long teeth and is similar to a pick comb but has a horizontal handle.

Tail comb – the tail end is great for sectioning, especially if you opt for a pin-tail design.

Teasing comb – its teeth are uniquely shaped so you can achieve back-combing without the damage. It adds volume and the tail end helps with sectioning.

BRUSHES

Detangler brush – great for all hair types, can be used on wet or dry hair and the flexible bristles help your hair become knot-free without damage.

Wet hairbrush – brushing your hair while wet can make it prone to breakages, however, if your hair is thick and curly it's better to brush it while wet or damp.

Cushion brush – for smoothing and taming.

Thermal brush – these come in round and paddle shapes and are made of a thermal material so while blow-drying, heat transfers to the brush and then onto your strands, speeding up drying time, smoothing and adding volume.

Boar bristle brush – their soft bristles glide through the hair, meaning less breakage, and they are great at smoothing and adding shine. They come in paddle, round or cushioned styles and are great for fine and thinning hair.

Nylon bristle brush – a synthetic bristle brush that helps detangle thick hair and reduce frizz.

Curved brush – lightweight, easy to use and often vented. Can be used on dry or wet hair. They're great for blow-drying as the vents help remove moisture fast.

Natural bristle brush – for anyone who wants the benefits of a boar bristle brush, but without the animal product. Great for vegans.

Mixed bristle brush – a mix of boar and nylon bristles, it's great at detangling long, thick hair.

Paddle brush – this brush has a wide base that helps smooth the hair and because of its size you can work on a bigger area. It's perfect for anyone with long straight hair.

Round brush – a good choice for blow-drying and styling loose waves. You can achieve volume at the root and curl under your hair to achieve waves or curls.

Scalp massager brush – great for maintaining a healthy scalp. You can use this while in the shower or on its own or after applying scalp products. It exfoliates, cleanses and stimulates the scalp.

HAIR STYLING ACCESSORIES

MICROFIBRE HAIR TOWEL

A microfibre hair towel is a highly absorbent and soft material in a shape that wraps perfectly around your hair. They're designed as an alternative to traditional towels as they offer reduced or heat-free drying, protect your hair from damage, extend your colour and combat frizz.

Because the material is so absorbent it means you can leave it on your hair to soak up the water after shampooing. It dries your hair well without the need for using a traditional towel to 'rub' it – it's this rubbing that causes friction and can result in damaged hair. And because it dries your hair well, you can reduce the amount of heat needed to fully dry your hair.

On my wash days I use a microfibre hair towel and I let it absorb the water while I'm doing my makeup. Once my makeup is done, I then add styling products and either air-dry or give it a low heat blast with a hairdryer. This routine really helps my bleached hair as heat is damaging, so I try to avoid heat as and when I can.

WATER SPRAY BOTTLE

I find having a water spray bottle on hand while doing hairstyles handy. It allows you to get your hair wet just enough without the need for washing it. It helps with styling and adding moisture back into the hair, which is one of our hair's basic needs. I use a water spray bottle to help with updos and braiding.

SILK PILLOW/HAIR WRAP

Every night while we sleep on cotton bed linen, we toss and turn, creating friction against our hair. This can cause breakage, frizz, split ends, dryness and thinner hair. Wearing a silk hair wrap or sleeping on a silk pillowcase combats this and really protects your locks. Silk is soft and non-absorbent, which means instead of causing friction your hair glides across it so it can retain its moisture and oils. A silk hair wrap also allows you to sleep while maintaining your hairstyle overnight – which is great if you're washing it less and want to avoid using heat too often. It can dramatically enhance the appearance of your hair.

> 'Wearing a silk bonnet and/or using a silk pillowcase when sleeping helps maintain my hair and reduces hair breakage. Any styles I have underneath can also be kept looking nice throughout the night'
> **BRIANA CAMPBELL (INFLUENCER)**

SECTIONING CLIPS/NO-CREASE CLIPS

If you're creating hairstyles or styling, it's a lot easier when you have sectioning clips at hand. You can clip aside the sections of hair you're not using for ease. No-crease clips are great to have in your kit so that when you're getting ready you can clip hair without adding a crease or kink to the look. They're also great when you need to tame your hair a certain way.

HAIR PINS

Bobby pins are essential when it comes to styling, as they hold hair in place. I'm always losing them, though – I'll buy a huge pack and suddenly they've disappeared. Who can relate? Not only are bobby pins handy, but U-shaped ones are great for updos and keeping buns secure.

HAIR BANDS

While hair bands are convenient, they can also be damaging, so it's good to be aware of how often you're using them, how you're taking them out and which styles you're doing with them. Ideally, you shouldn't pull your hair back too tight as this puts pressure on your hair follicles. Avoid sleeping with your hair tied up in a ponytail, as tossing and turning in the night can add more pressure to your hair roots, weakening them. Your hair is vulnerable when wet, so avoid tying your hair up as soon as you've washed it, too. Avoid hair bands with metal on, as these can pull on your hair and cause breakage.

Hair bands come in a lot of variations, so which should you choose?

No-slip – hair elastic coated in fabric, these are gentle on the hair and great for all hair types.

Spiral – the well-known Invisibobble, scientifically proven to cause less damage, less pain and fewer marks in your hair.

Scrunchies – these come in a variety of colours, prints, fabrics for accessorising ponytails and buns.

Silk – gentle on hair, help reduce creases and cause less damage.

Mini elastics – for securing small sections of hair, great for braiding. Can be damaging to hair if pulled out – my top tip is to cut them out of your hair or apply a hot curling iron to snap them.

Hook – these are great for securing updos and creating sleek ponytails. They're a no-slip hair band with a hook at each end. You hook one end into the hair, wrap the elastic around the hairstyle or ponytail and secure by attaching the other hook into the hair.

TOPSY TAIL

A hair tool that allows you to create multiple styles. It's easy to use and great for all hair types. It's got a tail end and the top is a flexible ring shape. It's perfect for achieving twist styles – for example, if you have a ponytail you put the tail end through the centre of the hair under the hair band, put the ponytail through the loop and pull it through.

HAIR DOUGHNUT

A hair doughnut is a circle of mesh that comes in a variety of colours and sizes that you can use to help create bun hairstyles. The longer your hair, the larger the doughnut size you will need. You put these through a ponytail and wrap the hair over the top, securing it with hair grips that go into the mesh.

VELCRO ROLLERS/HEATLESS CURLS

Heatless curls are great if you want to use less heat on your hair but still want to achieve volume and curls. Velcro rollers are easy to put in and come in different sizes, or you could try the TikTok viral overnight curls where you use a dressing gown tie and wrap your hair around it, sleeping in it overnight. That's a DIY way of doing it, but you can also buy a heatless curls kit, which comes with a satin tube that goes over your hair, then you wrap your hair around. They're comfortable to sleep in as you wrap your hair next to your ears, kind of like pigtails, leaving the back of your head free. However, these don't work so well on short hair.

HEATED TOOLS

If you do want to use heat on your hair to create your hairstyles there are numerous options to pick from.

Straighteners – for achieving sleek, straight hair with ease. However, they are multi-use as you can curl and wave hair with straighteners, too, using specific techniques that you will discover later in the book.

Blow-dryer brush – achieve a salon-worthy blow-dry at home with a blow-dryer brush. It's a 2-in-1 instead of using a hairdryer and round brush. You can create volume at the root easily and the mix of bristles helps detangle and smooth hair.

Curling tongs – these come in a variety of sizes and styles. You can find ones that clamp your hair or that you wrap your hair around. Ideally you want a curling tong that you can alter the heat setting on so you can change it according to your hair.

Waver – with a heated waver you can achieve consistent S-shaped waves all over the hair. They come in different sizes so you can find one to suit the length of your hair.

Hairdryer – we all know what a hairdryer does, try to find one with different attachments so it's versatile.

Heated rollers – for use on dry hair, hair rollers use a lower heat than a styling iron, but they take a while to apply. However, the curls tend to last longer as they've had longer to set. You can also achieve great volume at the root.

Heated brush – achieve smooth, sleek, straight hair with a heated brush.

Crimpers – these have a zig-zag plate that creates a zig-zag wave to the hair. It takes me back to my Spice Girls days, but crimpers are still great to use today. You can even use the technique of crimping your roots underneath your hair to create volume that holds.

My go-to brand for heat-styling tools is ghd. I've owned a pair of ghd straighteners since I was about 13 years old! My first ever pair lasted me around eight years, I remember having to get my dad to change the cable a few times to prolong their life. A lot has changed since then, especially with technology, which ghd incorporate into many of their tools. I also love that none of their tools go over 185 degrees with their heat – that is the maximum heat you should ever be putting on your hair, any higher and you're at risk of damage.

If you're looking for more affordable heated styling tools, look for ones with ceramic plates or even steam straighteners. Both are gentle on the hair and steam straighteners are less damaging.

HAIR ACCESSORIES

With these, you can have fun with different looks. Hair accessories allow you to jazz up a hairstyle like a simple ponytail or sleek straight hair. You can play around with hair clips or scrunchies that complement your outfit, or even use something like a claw clip to hold your updo in place.

Building a Haircare Routine

Everyone's hair is unique, therefore everyone's haircare routine will be different. What works for one person probably won't work for the next. For starters, we all have different hair types, porosity and density – I will go into these below – and we all treat our hair differently with the use of heat, styling and colour. Building a haircare routine can be a lot of trial and error and, like your skincare routine, sometimes you must change it up, as what once worked might not anymore. Our hair can go through changes, just like our skin, and be affected by pollution, nutrition, stress, lifestyle, medications, smoking, ageing, over-styling, cosmetic procedures and heredity factors.

'Just like we change our makeup and clothes seasonally, our haircare needs to as well. Consider using pre-shampoo treatments, especially in the summer months, to help retain moisture. R+Co Palm Springs is my personal favourite.'
HOLLIE BREWER, HAIR STYLIST

If you are struggling with your hair I'd always suggest seeking help from a professional stylist. I do regular check-ins with my stylist and colourist where we chat about my hair's health and products I should be using.

HAIR TEXTURE

When it comes to hair, there are four different types: straight, wavy, curly and coily. Essentially, it's all about your hair's curl pattern.

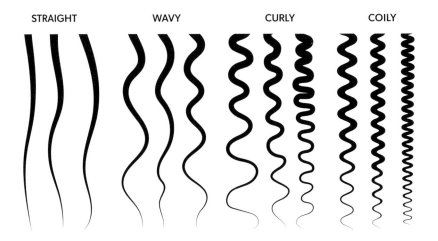

STRAIGHT   WAVY   CURLY   COILY

Knowing your hair type will help with your haircare routine. If you have tight coils, for example, you want to use products that define your curls. And if your hair has a soft wave, you want to use light products that enhance them and don't weigh the hair down.

HAIR POROSITY

Hair porosity and density are two other things to be mindful of when planning your haircare routine. Porosity is a measure of how well your hair can retain and absorb moisture. There are three levels of porosity – low, medium and high. The outside layer of the hair is known as the cuticle and how raised this is determines how porous your hair is.

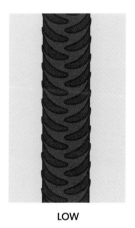

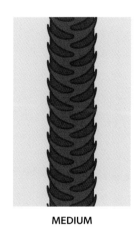

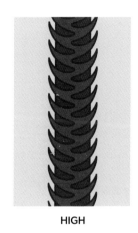

LOW **MEDIUM** **HIGH**

Several factors can affect the hair's porosity, such as genetics, the amount of heat you use, chemical processing and environmental factors. Knowing how porous your hair is will give you a better understanding of your hair and help you to choose the right products.

You can do a simple test at home to find your hair's porosity. Take some strands of hair from your brush or comb – make sure they are clean and free from product – drop them in a glass of water, then let them sit for a few minutes. If your hair is floating you have low porosity; if your hair is floating midway in the glass, it's medium; and if your hair sinks, it's high.

For more detailed information about afro, textured and curly hair, I'd recommend Charlotte Mensah's book, *Good Hair*.

WHAT DOES IT MEAN TO HAVE LOW, MEDIUM OR HIGH POROSITY?

Low porosity – the cuticles are overlapped and tightly packed together, which means water isn't easily absorbed, as well as other products like hair oils and conditioners that are used to inject moisture into the hair. You might find products sit on top of your hair and you can still feel them a few hours after you've applied them. To care for low-porosity hair you need to find products that have light ingredients that can easily penetrate, and apply them when your hair is wet and warm. Heat lifts the cuticle, allowing oils and moisture in – steam treatments can work wonders. Low-porosity hair naturally contains too much protein, so you want to avoid adding extra as this can cause the hair to become stiff and brittle, then break.

Medium porosity – the cuticle is slightly raised, so the hair allows in a steady flow of moisture that can be retained. This level of porosity stands up well to styling, colouring and chemicals and is the easiest to maintain. However, you need to be mindful of what you put this type of hair through, because it can easily increase in porosity. To maintain healthy hair, incorporate regular deep-conditioning and strengthening treatments into your routine for a balance of moisture and protein.

High porosity – the cuticle is wide open, so the hair allows moisture in but it doesn't stay long enough to nourish it. Highly porous hair can be genetic, but it can also result from chemical processing and styling like straightening, blow-drying and bleaching, all of which cause damage to the cuticles, causing them to lift or separate. If your hair is this level of porosity you might find it feels and looks dry, is prone to breakage, absorbs product quickly and tangles easily. With this porosity, you want to focus on reducing and reversing the damage to the cuticle and help your hair retain as much moisture as possible. Key ingredients to look for in products are coconut, avocado and olive oils as they help your strands retain moisture. Try to avoid heat, use a lower heat setting or air-dry the hair. Make sure you're always protecting the hair when styling and if you have coloured hair, high porosity means it's harder to retain colour. Use colour-protecting shampoos and conditioners to keep your colour vibrant for longer. Because the hair has many gaps in it from the raised cuticle, adding protein into your routine will reduce breakage and improve elasticity. Adding this strength and support will help structure your hair strands, improving texture. For added moisture, use a leave-in conditioner, and when applying a hair oil, do this last, as oils help seal moisture into the hair. You want to be gentle to your hair because it will be fragile with this level of porosity.

HAIR DENSITY

Density refers to the number of hairs on your head. Why do we need to know about it? I know, there's a lot to think about when it comes to your hair but it can all help with knowing which products to use. To figure out your hair's density, put your hair in a ponytail – if you can, of course – and measure the circumference of your tail where the hairband is. If it's less than 5 centimetres, you have low-density hair and if it's 10 centimetres or more you have high-density. Anything in between is medium. If you have short hair that you can't tie back, look at your scalp – the more your scalp is seen through your hair, the lower the density.

It's also good to know how thick each individual strand is. You could have thick hair strands but a low density. A trick for seeing the thickness of your hair is to measure it next to a strand of thread. If your hair is thinner than the thread, it's thin, if it's thicker than the thread, it's thick.

Low density – you want to avoid heavy products that will weigh your hair down; opt for ones that offer volumising. Styles that offer volume at the root will give you the appearance of thicker hair.

Medium density – your hair is in the middle, you won't need to do much to achieve volume. Experiment with hairstyles and try to maintain healthy locks.

High density – you might need heavy styling products to be able to tame your mane. Half-up hairstyles could work well to tie back some of the bulk and if there is too much of your hair, you could always get a stylist to add in layers, as this thins its appearance.

Unfortunately, hair density is genetic and you cannot change the number of hair follicles you have. If you have low-density hair and lack hair in specific areas, you could opt for a hair transplant to even out growth.

HAIR ELASTICITY

The final thing to take note of with your hair is its elasticity – its natural stretch – because hair elasticity can affect your hair in lots of different ways: how easy it is to manage, how healthy it is and its shine. Hairs are made up of protein (keratin) and moisture and it's the protein that helps maintain its elasticity that gives your strands their structure and strength.

There's a really easy test you can do to determine the elasticity of your hair: the stretch test.

1. With your hair wet, select a strand and hold it at the root to avoid pulling it out.

2. With your other hand, gently stretch the hair, then release. If it stretches and returns to its original length your elasticity is good.

3. If your hair:

   - doesn't stretch or it breaks, it lacks moisture, meaning you have low elasticity.

   - stretches A LOT but doesn't return back to its original form (maybe it feels mushy between your fingers), it lacks protein and therefore has high elasticity.

   - stretches and breaks, it's lacking both protein and moisture.

So now you've done the tests and you've figured out your hair type, you can start to build a care routine to give it what it needs.

YOUR ROUTINE

Here's a basic guide to a haircare routine that you can build from and mould to suit your hair and its needs, followed by some great tips I want to share with you all.

STEP 1: CLEANSING

A haircare routine always starts with cleansing using shampoo. The focus of a shampoo is to cleanse your roots and scalp of dirt, oil and product build-up, so it's important to know your scalp type before picking a shampoo. For example, if you're prone to oily roots you may need a shampoo that focuses on deep cleansing over moisturising. Or if your scalp is tight and dry, you might want to opt for a moisturising shampoo. When shampooing you only need a small, coin-sized amount to lather up and massage into your roots and scalp.

Essentially, shampoo is for your roots and scalp and masks or conditioners are for your ends, so treat them both separately.

TYPES OF SHAMPOO:

Regular everyday – one that isn't specific to one's hair needs, it just gently cleanses.

Clarifying – this goes a lot further than your everyday shampoo, it deep cleanses and is great for product build-up or oily roots. Clarifying shampoos contain sulphates, which most people try to avoid as they can be drying and harsh, but this is the best type of shampoo for cleansing and removing oils.

Thickening – formulated to add body and fullness to the hair while gently cleansing, strengthening and protecting it from future breakage. Great for fine hair.

Volumising – great for fine hair, as it focuses on volume by cleansing while lifting hair from the root. It leaves the hair visibly fuller.

Strengthening – for damaged hair that may be suffering from breakage. A repairing shampoo focuses on strengthening as well as cleansing, to help prevent further breakages and split ends. If the damage is extreme you might look for a bond-building repair shampoo. This type of shampoo has a bond-building technology within its formula to shield the weakened bonds from further damage.

Colour-treated hair – this will keep coloured hair looking vibrant for longer. Look for one that's sulphate-free for semi-permanent hair colours. These types of shampoo also have added benefits for the hair, such as repairing.

Dandruff – these shampoos work best at getting rid of dandruff and can be purchased with a prescription strength. They contain an active ingredient called ketoconazole, which is an anti-fungal medicine and works by treating the underlying cause of dandruff.

Moisturising – if your hair is feeling dry, a moisturising shampoo will focus on cleansing but also nourishing and rehydrating the hair.

Curly hair – these shampoos have been specifically formulated for curly hair so that they cleanse but keep your curls hydrated.

Toning – usually a purple or silver shampoo (for blondes) but you can find blue ones on the market (for brunettes). They're aimed at cleansing the hair but also moisturising, brightening and neutralising brassy tones.

With so many shampoo brands on the market it can be tricky to choose what's right for you. Be conscious of the ingredients and if it's right for your hair. If you want to be more environmentally conscious you can now find shampoo bars, which are a great alternative to buying plastic shampoo bottles. Some brands even offer refills.

Ever heard of a double shampoo? It's where you pre-cleanse your hair before shampooing it. It's kind of like how you would double cleanse in your skincare routine. The first cleanse removes dirt, impurities and any product build-up, the second cleanses and nourishes. Double shampooing might not be right for everyone's hair type, though, it totally depends on the condition of your hair and scalp. For example, if your hair is extremely damaged and fragile, a double shampoo might be too much.

You don't need to double shampoo all the time. For my own bleached hair, which is fragile, I tend to do a double shampoo if I'm trying to fade a semi-permanent hair colour faster or if my hair has got a lot of product build-up, such as when I've worn a lot of hair gel or hairspay for an updo style. It's not often, I'd say maybe twice a month. If you find double shampooing doesn't work for you, you could opt for a clarifying shampoo instead on the odd occasion where you feel like your hair needs it.

STEP 2: HAIR MASK

Hair masks are especially great for dry or damaged hair as they act as an intense, deep treatment, but all hair types can benefit, as masks are formulated with rich ingredients such as keratin, vitamins and oils. When looking for a hair mask, find one specific for your hair's needs – such as hydrating, repairing or strengthening – and find one suitable for your hair type. There are lots on the market aimed at fine to thick hair.

A hair mask should be used before your conditioner, and if you're not using one in your routine, you should be! They deeply nourish the hair and have so many added benefits to meet all your hair concerns. They go deeper than a conditioner. Applying them after a shampoo is key as shampooing opens up the hair follicle so the ingredients will penetrate. Limit how often you apply a hair mask to once a week and find ones that you leave on from three minutes to overnight. Don't forget to comb it through so your hair is evenly coated.

STEP 3: CONDITIONER

Conditioner comes next, and its purpose is to improve the texture and feel of your hair, along with hydrating, adding shine and making it more manageable for you to style. It also adds a protective layer to your hair strands, protecting them against the environment and heat styling.

When you use conditioner, do not apply it to the scalp. You want to focus on your mid-length hair, down to the ends. I recommend combing it through using a wide-tooth comb to make sure your hair is evenly coated. A conditioner isn't left on for as long as a hair mask – around three minutes is usually the average.

You should always use a conditioner after shampooing, and if you opt for a hair mask, make sure the conditioner is applied after. This is because your conditioner is adding that protective layer, so if you apply a hair mask after your conditioner it won't be able to penetrate fully and nourish your hair.

When it comes to picking a conditioner, unlike shampoo your conditioner needs to be selected according to your actual hair, over your scalp. For example, your scalp might be oily, but the ends of your hair dry; therefore you'd choose a clarifying shampoo specific to your scalp's needs and a hydrating conditioner for your ends.

There are a variety of different conditioners on the market, just like shampoos. From hydrating, volumising and strengthening to ones aimed at curly or straight hair.

Hydrating – focuses on adding moisture back into the hair, as well as shine and smoothness.

Volumising – formulated for fine, flat hair to promote body and volume while nourishing and smoothing without weighing the hair down.

Strengthening – focuses on repairing and nourishing damaged and weak hair while adding back moisture and leaving the hair smooth, shiny and healthy-looking.

Balancing – formulated to achieve naturally balanced, healthy hair. Not too moisturising, but it won't dry your hair out and works well on most hair types.

Smoothing – focuses on taming frizzy hair, this is protecting and nourishing and leaves hair feeling smoother and more manageable.

Colour-protecting – keeps your colour vibrant for longer while nourishing, protecting and adding shine.

Thickening – formulated to add volume while it nourishes, leaving the illusion of hair with fuller body and bounce.

Purifying – focuses on nourishing, smoothing and restoring hair while cleansing ends free of impurities and product build-up so hair isn't weighed down.

Curl – a super-hydrating formula that helps moisturise and detangle curls without weighing them down.

Toning – comes as a purple or silver conditioner that focuses on neutralising brassy tones on blonde hair while also moisturising and leaving hair soft and sleek. You can also find blue conditioners that neutralise unwanted brassy tones in brunette hair.

A top tip from my hairdresser, Hollie Brewer, is: 'I recommend replacing your conditioner with a hair mask once a week, I get a lot of clients who find it hard to allow the extra time in their routine so my go-to product tends to be Davines, the Circle Chronicles range. Something for everyone! Plus the brand is sustainable!'

STEP 4: LEAVE-IN TREATMENTS

Leave-in products are lightweight formulas that provide the hair with extra moisture to help protect from damage. They can be found as leave-in conditioners or leave-in treatments and you will be able to find one specific to your hair's needs. These are applied to damp, towel-dried hair and left in, you do not rinse them out like a shampoo/hair mask/conditioner.

How often should you apply a leave-in? Every time you wash your hair and on those in-between hair wash days where you feel like your hair needs some extra hydration. You won't need to use a lot as a little goes a long way, and you won't harm your hair by protecting it with a leave-in.

You'll find most leave-in products to be super-hydrating, and depending on which product you pick, they can also detangle, smooth the hair, seal split ends, protect, minimise the appearance of damage, add shine and reduce frizz.

Leave-in products can be found as sprays, mists, creams or balms and are beneficial for all hair types. If you have fine hair, a mist works well as it won't weigh down the hair, and for thick hair, go for a cream or balm with a thicker texture. If you have curly hair, hydration is key for achieving bouncy, defined curls. You will want a light leave-in formula so it doesn't weigh down your curls; a spray would work well.

If you have bleached hair like mine, investing in K18 can completely transform your hair. K18 is a leave-in treatment mask for all hair types that clinically reverses damage in 4 minutes. The patented peptide technology works to repair damage from bleach, colour, chemical services and heat – restoring strength, softness, smoothness and bounce to hair. I use this every 5–6 washes straight after shampooing and leave it in. This replaces my in-shower mask and conditioner and I just follow up with a leave-in conditioner and the rest of my haircare routine.

How often should you apply a leave-in? Every time you wash your hair! You won't need to use a lot, as a little goes a long way, but it doesn't harm your hair by protecting it with a leave-in.

STEP 5: HAIR OILS AND SERUMS

You can apply hair oils and serums on damp or dry hair. As previously mentioned, applying on damp hair is the most effective as our hair is more absorbent when wet. Hair oils and serums are another way of strengthening our locks, taming frizz and hydrating.

STEP 6: STYLING CREAMS AND MOUSSE

Once you've applied your leave-in product and oils, you're ready to start styling. If you're using a blow-dry cream or wanting volume from a mousse, then you'd apply this as your next step.

STEP 7: HEAT PROTECT

Using heat on your hair? Never forget this step! A heat-protecting spray is going to prevent heat damage, so it's crucial you apply it.

STEP 8: BLOW-DRYING AND AIR-DRYING

I guess it depends how much time we all have, but once your hair is dry, you're ready to style.

STEP 9: STYLING AND FINISHING

Everyone styles their hair in a way that's unique to them so we all use different products in this final step. You might be straightening your hair, so apply a styling cream or oil for extra smoothness and shine. If you're curling your hair, you might be grabbing your hold spray, or if you're wanting a beachy and textured finish, spritz a beach spray over your locks.

Now you've got a basic step-by-step routine for your hair-wash days you can start to look into what your hair needs and form your routine to suit. On average everyone washes their hair every 2–3 days, so in between your wash days start from step 4 of your haircare routine – if your hair needs extra moisture from a leave-in product – and then move on to your hair oils, heat-protecting and styling. And remember, as Hollie Brewer says, 'when using any product make sure you follow the instructions for best results.'

HAIRCARE TIPS

As well as the basic routine, I have some great haircare tips and hacks to share with you all that are super-useful to know about, so take note!

1. **Never go to bed with wet hair**

This is something I did for years when I was younger. I'm sure we've all been there and I definitely learned the hard way because of the breakage I endured from sleeping with my hair wet. Your hair is most fragile when wet, so tossing and turning in the night is going to lead to breakage.

2. **Don't overload on hair products**

Use minimal product and it won't weigh your hair down or lead to product build-up. We don't need to apply 10 different products to our hair, as long as we're giving it what it needs, we could use just one product that has a multitude of benefits.

3. **Avoid using hot water on your hair**

Opt for lukewarm water instead, as hot water can cause stress on your hair that can lead to breakage. If you can, finish your hair wash with cold water to seal the follicles. Briana Campbell says, 'I prefer to use warm or cool water on my hair to maintain my curls. Hot water can cause our hair to lose its natural moisture and makes it feel thinner. Cold water helps retain that hydration and helps keep my curls defined and bouncy.'

4. **Take breaks between hairstyles**

Another thing that puts stress on your hair is doing the same style over and over. For example, if you wear a ponytail every day, you are putting stress on the same place on your hair strands and this can lead to breakage. Give your hair a break or switch things up, and try a different style.

5. **Protect your hair from the sun**

Sun exposure can dry your hair out, especially if it's colour-treated or bleached. Make sure to either wear a hat, cover up or use a UV hairspray for extra protection.

6. **Trim your split ends and get regular trims**

It's important to keep on top of split ends, so they don't keep splitting or cause breakage. You can trim your split ends at home, they're really easy to spot, or book a regular trim every 6–8 weeks.

7. **Turn your hot tools onto a low or medium setting**

It can be tempting to turn your straighteners on to the highest heat setting to style your hair, but heat is damaging and you can usually style your hair just as well with a lower heat setting, which will be a lot kinder to it.

8. **Wet your hair before swimming**

Your hair is absorbent, so if you wet it with clean water before going into the ocean or a swimming pool, it will already be saturated and won't be able to absorb much more water, thus protecting it.

9. **Apply a water-resistant mask before swimming**

If you prefer, you can be prepared with a water-resistant conditioner or mask. Apply this to damp hair and it adds a protective layer that helps protect it from the drying and damaging effects of chlorinated and salt water.

10. **Don't forget to clean your hairbrush**

Hairbrushes should be cleaned often as product can build up in your brush, which can lead to your hair becoming greasy. Simply, remove the hair from the brush, then soak it in hot water and clarifying shampoo.

11. **Don't spray perfume on your hair**

Perfumes have a high concentration of alcohol, so if you're spritzing your go-to perfume all over your hair every day, over time it can cause dehydration, which can lead to damage.

12. **Eat healthily**

Eating protein isn't just good for the body, it's also great for the hair. If you eat nutritious foods, they promote stronger, healthier hair. Eggs, salmon, berries and nuts are great as they contain high amounts of protein and omega-3 fats.

13. Tame your flyaways

A technique I like to use to tame flyaways is to spray hairspray on my hands then carefully pat down any stray hairs. It keeps them in place without the crunchy feel and look or too much product.

14. Don't blow-dry until your hair is around 75% dry

Remember your hair is wet when you blow-dry and hairdriers are hot. If you blow-dry after towel drying, the water particles in your hair will heat up, and we all know heat is damaging. Use a microfibre hair towel – I have one available from Sophie Hannah Hair – which will absorb a lot of the water, then when your hair is around 75% dry, you can blow-dry.

15. Give your hair a break

If you're not going anywhere, resist applying heat or washing it for a day or a few days. This is great if your hair is damaged. Briana Campbell says, 'I try to avoid heat as much as possible – that includes blow-drying and straightening – to prevent heat damage and curl destruction. I only straighten my hair a max of four times a year, but I try to keep it under three. When I do apply heat, I make sure to add a heat protectant to all of my hair beforehand

16. Massage your scalp!

Massaging your scalp increases blood circulation and can promote hair growth. Try doing it for five minutes daily – consistency is key here, so try a routine you can stick to.

17. Manage stress

Easier said than done, stress is a normal part of life. But stress can affect your hair and scalp and lead to thinning or shedding hair. There are many ways we can manage stress, which is good for mental and physical health too; try exercise, meditation, mindfulness apps, setting aside 'me' time. I like to use the Calm app, as it centres me and leaves me feeling fully relaxed.

Hair Colour

As you know, I'm constantly switching up my hair colour; I think I've been every colour of the rainbow by now. I've been doing this for over 14 years, it's a way for me to get creative and experiment and it's just fun. Who's with me? My hair is a part of my style, identity and it reflects my outgoing personality. You only live once, if you want coloured hair, go for it!

For most of us that want to achieve vibrant, bright colours, it does require lifting our hair to a level 9/10 on the dark to light scale, which can mean we need to turn to bleach. That's the only downside to having coloured hair, what you must put it through. You will most likely have bad days, like me, where your hair snaps off from bleach, and it's hard work growing it back, but if your hair is a part of you, I think it's worth it. I don't feel like myself if I haven't got coloured hair, and my freshly bleached hair never stays blonde for long.

If you do want to switch up your colour but maybe you are dark, brunette or auburn, if you look for a highly pigmented dye it can either offer your hair a tint or a deep, rich result.

Semi-permanent colours are not damaging to the hair, it's only bleaching that is. You can switch up your colour with semi-permanent dyes as often as you like, as most on the market do not contain any damaging harsh chemicals . Essentially, all that semi-permanent hair colour does is deposit colour molecules to the cuticle layer, coating the outside of each strand. This type of dye fades with each wash, so it's a great choice if you love to switch up your colour often.

When looking for a semi-permanent hair dye, look for ones that are free from PPD (paraphenylenediamine), which is a known allergen, ammonia and resorcinol as these can be toxic or damaging, and instead offer ingredients that are going to benefit and nourish your hair. I actually have my own brand of semi-permanent hair colours called Sophie Hannah Hair, which have been formulated with added benefits to repair, strengthen and nourish the hair, as well as colouring it.

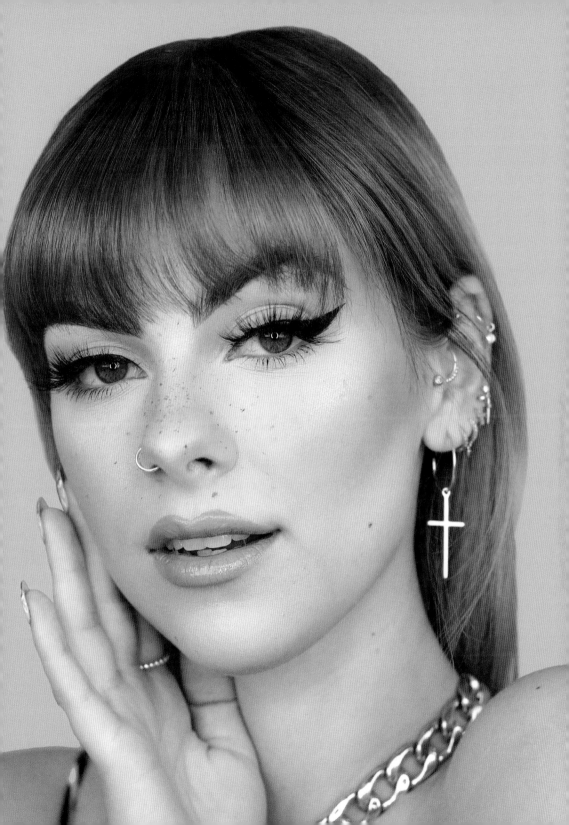

HOW TO TAKE CARE OF COLOURED HAIR

If you're going to all the effort of colouring your hair, you're going to want to take extra good care of it, especially because most of the time it might have been pre-bleached. Over years of dyeing my hair, I've trialled lots of different ways to help my colour last and take care of my hair, so I'm going to pass these on to you.

1. Don't shampoo after using a semi-permanent hair colour
Rinse your hair using cool water, this will help lock the colour in as using hot water opens the hair's cuticle and the dye you just spent 20 minutes applying can escape during the rinse.

2. Wait three days before you wash your hair
Avoid washing your hair for three days after colouring it, as that way you'll ensure the colour is locked in and lasts longer. It can take a few days after dyeing for your hair's cuticles to close and trap in the dye.

3. Don't wash your hair often
People always say to me, your hair colour is lasting so long, but that's because I avoid washing my hair too often. Every time you wash it, your semi-permanent colour will fade.

4. Wash your hair separately
I'm a lover of a hot steamy bath or shower, but washing your hair in that temperature is going to make your colour fade fast. Wash your hair separately with cool water.

5. Limit heat styling
Heat styling opens the hair cuticles, so just like washing in hot water, your colour will fade faster. Protect your hair with a heat-protecting spray if you are going to use heat, or try heatless hairstyles or curls.

6.

Protect your colour from the sun

The sun is not your friend if you have coloured hair; exposure to the sun can fade it, so make sure to either cover up or protect hair using a UV spray.

7.

Use sulphate-free shampoo and conditioner

Sulphates strip the hair of its natural oils and moisture and if it's stripping that out, it's also going to strip your colour. You can find sulphate-free shampoos and conditioners for your specific hair needs or opt for a colour-protecting range. You don't need to avoid sulphate-free products, though, as these tend to be great for cleansing and if you have oily roots or product build-up. However, if you want your semi-permanent colour to last longer, it's a good tip to remember.

8.

Add your hair colour to your conditioner

Want to keep your hair vibrant for longer and the colour topped up? Mix a small amount into your go-to conditioner every time or every few times you wash your hair.

9.

Use leave-in treatments

Leave-in treatments will protect your colour when styling, and coloured and chemically treated hair needs extra hydration and protection. Find a leave-in product that has a multitude of benefits, such as UV protection.

10.

Avoid chlorine and salt water

Both of these will instantly strip the colour out of your hair, so make sure you coat your hair in a water-resistant mask before swimming.

11.

Get regular trims

Dead, split ends won't hold colour and will fade fast, so to keep your colour looking fresh from root to tip, get regular trims.

APPLYING HAIR COLOUR

Applying semi-permanent or even permanent hair colour takes a little practice, but with the right tools and application you can achieve some amazing looks. Always use gloves to prevent staining on your hands or nails, and it's helpful to use a dye kit that comes with a bowl and brush, as this will help you achieve a consistent, even application.

If I'm applying a full head of colour, I always start at the back, underneath, and work my way to the front, starting with the roots, then dye the lengths of my hair. I use this technique even if I'm only dyeing small sections.

One thing that helps me a lot when dyeing my hair is working in sections. Divide up your hair before you start applying your colour – you can use clips for this – which will help keep the application neat, and if you are applying multiple colours it keeps them separated during the process while the colour works into your hair.

If you do get any colour on your skin or scalp this can be removed during application or after. If you're using a pigmented colour like red or blue that could cause staining on the skin, I'd recommended wiping it off your skin as soon as possible. However, with a wash or two the staining will fade from your skin and using a scalp massager can help remove any colour that's lingered on your scalp. Or if you have any Vaseline handy, apply some along the edge of your hairline before you start dyeing, as it creates a barrier so the dye doesn't penetrate and stain.

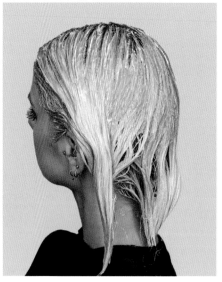
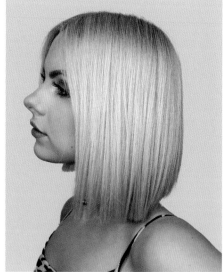

HAIR COLOUR INSPIRATION

When it comes to dyeing my hair I'm always faced with 'what colour shall I do next?' and 'how should I dye it?'. The possibilities are endless when you're experimenting with hair colour, that's the fun of it! So to help you out the next time you want to dye your hair, I thought I'd put together a bunch of ideas to inspire you.

ONE COLOUR

If you don't want to put too much effort into the process, why not just pick one colour – it could be neon, pastel or something super vibrant. Picking one colour makes it a lot easier to maintain, too, as you can pop the dye into your conditioner and keep it topped up when washing.

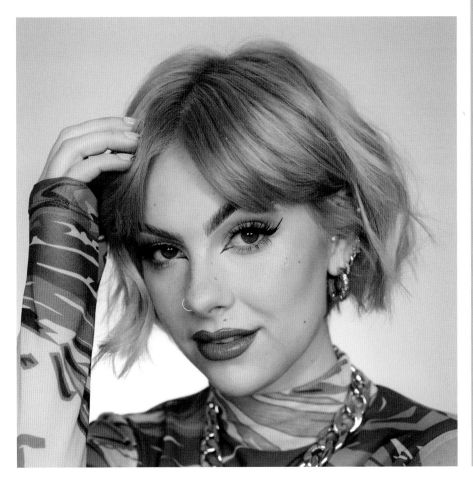

MONEY PIECE

This is a very popular way of adding a pop of colour into your look and it also means you don't need to bleach your whole head to achieve it. Money piece is where you colour two sections of hair at the front to add framing to your face. You can do this with one colour or even ombre a few together. If you like the money piece look but want more hair coloured, you can bring the sections round to your ears and underneath the back of your hair.

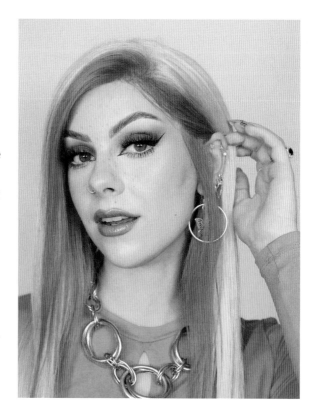

GRADIENT

I love a gradient look because of the many different combinations you can try. I find a gradient look works best by starting with your darkest shade at the root and as you work your way down to the tip, you blend it into a lighter shade(s). When creating an ombre look you can select as many colours as you want. I find picking 2–3 works well, but the longer your hair, the more you can work with.

When applying, it's best to work in sections and start with your root colour. Use a brush, then place small sections of hair in between your index and middle finger and drag the colour down to achieve a smooth blend. Make sure you slightly overlap each shade and use the index and middle finger technique to blend between the colours.

Great colour combinations for an ombre look are:

Red > orange > yellow   Turquoise > lime

Dark purple > pink   Blue > green

Dark purple > silver   Blue > purple > red

Purple > blue   Pink > yellow

There are no rules when it comes to hair colour, though, so if you want to experiment doing a lighter shade at the root and graduating to a darker shade on the tips, go for it! I've seen some cool looks on Pinterest where people have done this.

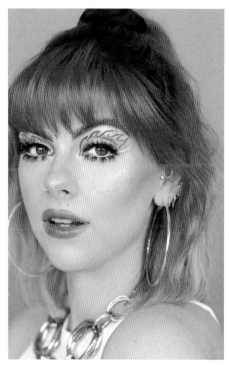 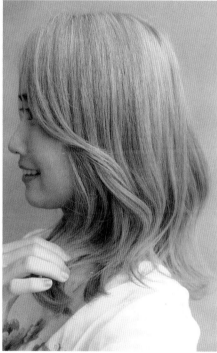

SPLIT HAIR

Can't pick one colour? Why not choose two?! I love a split-hair look and it's super-easy to do as long as you can evenly part your hair down the centre. Some great colour combinations for a split hair look are:

Blue and green

Purple and blue

Black and a colour

Pink and green

Pink and purple

Blonde and a colour

Orange and pink

Purple and turquoise

Or if you're wanting more than two colours you could pick four and do a split hair look, but each side is a gradient of two colours. I've done this a few times before and it looks eye-catching.

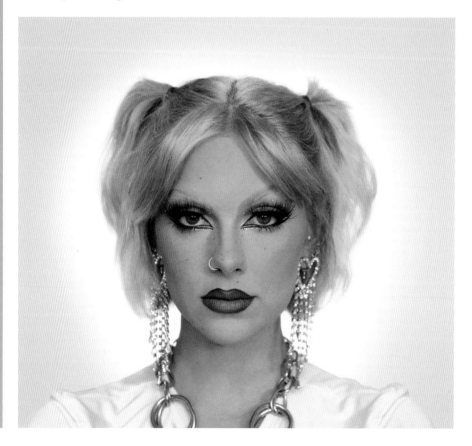

TIPS

Another way to add some colour into your locks is to just dye the tips. This is great if you've got mid-dark hair, as for bright vibrant tips you'd only have to bleach the very ends. Coloured tips look great on every hair colour and length. You might have dark brown hair and go for red tips, or have bleach-blonde hair and do bright blue tips!

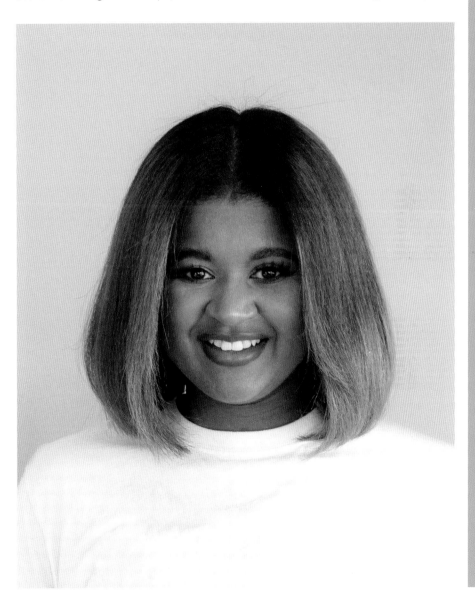

RAINBOW

Rainbow hair is the most colourful and vibrant of them all and I love the fact that there are so many different variations you can create.

Rainbow gradient – start with red at the top and blend down through each colour. You could do this all over your hair or even just the two money pieces.

Hidden rainbow hair – colour a section through the back of your hair, in the centre, so it's hidden under your top layer, sandwiched between the top and underneath. Colour in sections from left to right, starting with red and working your way through the colours of the rainbow.

Multi-rainbow – you could divide your hair into small sections all over and apply every colour of the rainbow individually on each separate section. The overall look will be multi-coloured streaks that all blend together.

Split-hair rainbow – another option is to split your hair down the middle and on one side apply a gradient of red into orange into yellow, and on the other a gradient of purple into blue into green.

Rainbow fringe – if you have a fringe you want to highlight you could add a rainbow gradient to that or apply rainbow colours in small sections from left to right.

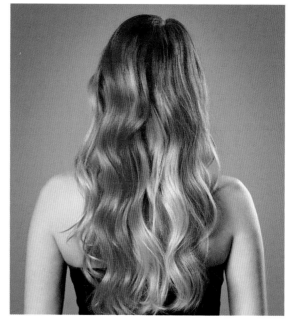

UNDERNEATH COLOUR

Instead of splitting your hair down the centre, why not split it across – like if you were doing a half-up, half-down hairstyle. Keep the top in your natural hair colour or bleached and the underneath layer a block colour. When you style your hair wavy, the underneath colour will peep through and if you wear your hair in a ponytail you will see the bold split.

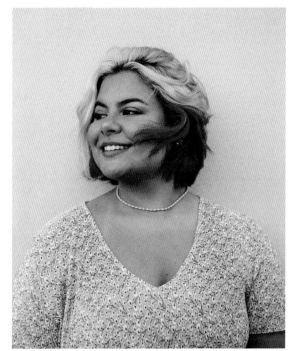

HIDDEN HAIR COLOUR

Adding on from hidden rainbow hair, instead of picking rainbow colours you could do a single colour instead and keep it hidden within the back section of your hair, sandwiched between the top and underneath layers.

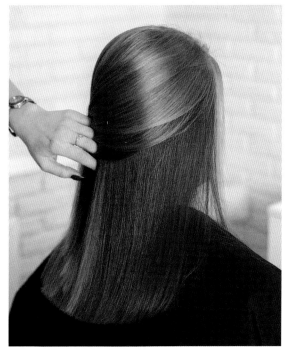

PATTERNS

Feeling extra creative? Why not experiment with a few colours and create a pattern out of the application. If you have a bleached buzzcut you could paint on stars, flames, hearts, or even swirls for a really bold, eye-catching look. Or if your hair is longer you could apply the dye in dots or make stencils in different shapes, then use as a template over the hair and fill in with colour.

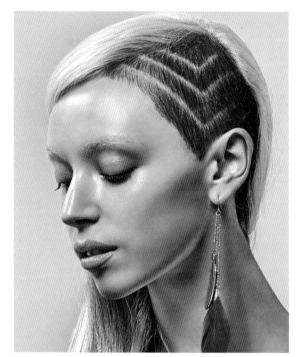

UNICORN

And finally, unicorn hair! Which is pretty much multi-pastel colours: lilac, ice blue, mint green, baby pink. That colour palette gives all the unicorn vibes; when it comes to the application apply the colours randomly to small sections all over your hair.

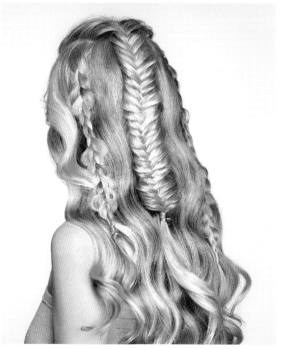

REMOVING SEMI-PERMANENT HAIR COLOUR

A question I get asked a lot is how I remove my semi-permanent colours. I've tried and tested a lot of different methods over the years and if I'm honest, they've all been quite damaging. I've tried semi-permanent colour removers from brands that say they are ammonia and damage-free but in fact they did damage my hair because they had other ingredients within their formulas or some colour removers that were essentially just as harsh as bleaching. If you have bleached hair, you'll know you shouldn't really be bleaching over already bleached hair more than once as it can cause extreme damage.

When trying to remove semi-permanent colour from the hair, Hollie Brewer always recommends seeing a professional colourist. 'The integrity of your hair is most important and needs to be done as safely as possible. There are some things you can do at home as a natural process like using baking powder and shampoo that can help to break down SOME colour molecules.'

So here are a few DIY tips you can attempt that do work fairly well, but it totally depends on how vibrant your hair colour is beforehand and what shade you are.

1. **Wash your hair... a lot!**
This is how I remove a lot of my semi-permanent hair colours. I am patient and wait for the colour to fade gradually with every wash, then when it's around 70–80% faded I will get a strong clarifying shampoo (that contains sulphates) and shampoo my hair numerous times in one go. I make sure the water is hot (not boiling) as this opens the hair follicle and allows colour to escape and I shampoo all my hair – roots to tips. After doing this a few times, I follow up with an intense, deep-conditioning hair mask. This technique will work for most semi-permanent colours, however, it won't completely budge blues and greens.

2. **Vitamin C or bicarbonate of soda and anti-dandruff or clarifying shampoo**
Crush a few vitamin C tablets to turn them into powder or buy powdered vitamin C and mix with a drop of anti-dandruff shampoo until it turns into a foam mixture. Apply on wet hair as you would normal shampoo, but concentrate on the roots down to the tips of the hair. Lather it up like a

normal shampoo then pop your hair in a shower cap and leave for around 45 minutes. Follow up with a deep-conditioning hair mask because this will dry your hair out. Another option is to mix bicarbonate of soda with anti-dandruff shampoo instead of vitamin C and let it sit on the hair for around 20 minutes. Again, you will want to follow up with a deep-conditioning hair mask. This technique works best on hair colour that's pretty much faded out and maybe you're left with a pastel hue or a tint. It won't budge blues and greens much though – trust me, I've tried!

3. Detergent

Before shampooing your hair, grab your dishwashing detergent from your kitchen and apply it to your hair as you would shampoo. Lather it up, rinse and follow up with your normal shampoo; hair mask and/or conditioner. It works so well because of all the sulphates in the formula. Super-simple, but again, it can be drying and probably won't budge the blues and greens.

4. Vinegar

Using vinegar is probably the least-damaging method of removing semi-permanent hair colour. It might not strip all the colour out at once so you might need to repeat it a few times. Mix together two cups of water and half a cup of white vinegar. Shampoo your hair as normal, rinse and towel dry. Apply the water and vinegar mix onto the hair, pop over a shower cap and leave it on for about 20 minutes. You can follow up with another shampoo afterwards and the rest of your haircare routine.

There are other methods, but these are the least-damaging and will avoid bleach or lightening and lifting the hair. In an ideal world, be patient and let the colour fade naturally over time, but if you can't be patient, you can utilise your coloured hair and still change shades. Think of your hair like mixing paints; if you put a red dye over faded blue hair, it'll turn purple, or if you put yellow over faded blue it'll turn green. If you can avoid stripping your faded colour out of your hair completely, you will cause no damage. A useful tip I learned about hair colour and changing shades was to use a colour wheel.

It's a simple theory; knowing the colour wheel will help with changing up your colour and even neutralising unwanted tones. For example, with blonde or bleached hair, purple shampoo neutralises unwanted yellow tones. You can see on the wheel that purple is opposite yellow, while blue toners cancel out orange and green cancels out red. This theory is used by hairdressers when colour correcting, but we can apply this at home too.

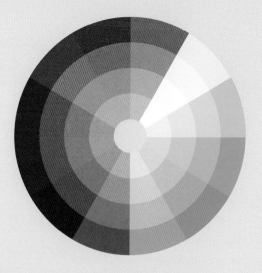

If you're a fellow hair colourer you'll know that blues and greens cause staining and linger on the hair for ages! Blue hair is a commitment because of this. It's just impossible to get out of your hair without bleaching and causing further damage. However, there are a few things you can do.

First is to fade your blue as much as possible – it will likely go to a mint-green hue. Refer to your colour wheel – opposite blue/green on the spectrum is orange/red/pink. Instead of trying a damaging method for removing the blue, you can neutralise it by making your own toner. Dilute an orange/red/pink dye (depending on what shade of faded blue/green you have) with conditioner and massage into your hair. You will want to do a strand test first in case the mixture is too pigmented. Apply, keep an eye on it, then rinse. You can repeat this step as often as you need to. But if you've got the toner to just the right shade, it will neutralise the faded blue/green. I've tried this many times and it works so well. It gives me a cleaner base to then try a new colour.

Another way I've tried to remove faded green from my hair is to dye my hair with a really pigmented shade of the opposite colour. So, for faded green I created a gradient of pigmented magenta into red, into orange. When this faded, my hair went back blonde, because the colour neutralised the leftover green.

If you don't fancy trying this method, you could be clever about which colours you pick next by working your way around the colour wheel. It's much easier transitioning your hair colour to a shade next to it on the wheel than jumping to the opposite side. For example, if you have green hair, the next colour you could go would be blue. Then you can easily change that to purple, then purple to red, red to orange and so on.

Wigs

Don't fancy getting into the world of bleach but still want to try vibrant, bold colours? Or maybe you want to try out a new hairstyle before taking the plunge? Why not turn to wigs? I love wearing wigs, they're a great way to switch up your look without any long-term effects.

Wearing a wig is something else I have experimented with over the years, mainly because I have short bobbed hair and it allows me to add length. I always opt for human hair over synthetic, because I like the versatility of being able to dye it, tone it and style it. However, human hair wigs can be pricey, so synthetic wigs can be a great alternative. Find one that's already coloured and to which you can apply heat, so you can style them.

When buying a human hair wig, depending on where you're shopping you will get to choose specific things such as colour, lace style, lace size, hair length, hair density, cap size, baby hairs, hair part and lace colour. Which options you pick will determine the price of the wig.

Wigs come in many styles, but I prefer either a lace front or full lace. Lace fronts are cheaper than full-lace wigs, however full-lace are more versatile because they can be worn in different hairstyles. With a lace-front wig, often with certain hairstyles you might see the cap of the wig showing through the hair – for example, with a half-up, half-down hairstyle.

How I 'install' my wigs is something I often get asked. Sometimes I don't do it properly if I know I'm going to wear a hat or headband that covers the hairline, however if the hairline is out, I use this technique, which keeps my wig in place all day, or even for a few days.

- Prep your hair by putting it into two French braids – if your hair is long enough to do so. If not, twist two strands and add in hair each time you twist. Do this in small sections from the front of your hair to the back. Essentially you want to style your hair as flat against your head as possible. Once you've done this, place a wig cap over the top – try to opt for one closest to your skin tone.

- Clean your hairline; you want to install your wig before doing your makeup.

- Position your wig before you apply adhesives. Roughly put your wig on and line it up to where you want your hairline to start. Then trim the lace and, if needed, around your ears for a better fit. Take it off and put it to the side.

- The next step is gluing down the wig cap. I like to use got2b Glued Blasting Freeze Spray for this. Pull your wig cap down over your ears and to just above your brows. Taking your freeze spray, hold it close to your head and spray along the edge of your hairline, from ear to ear. Smooth out with your finger and use a hairdryer to speed up drying of the spray.

- Before trimming around the edge of the lace, carefully cut a hole where your ears are and poke them through the lace. Then taking your freeze spray again, spray around the front edge of your ears.

- Once the freeze spray has dried, carefully take scissors and cut the lace around the edge of your hairline.

- To blend the wig cap into your skin, take your foundation and apply on top of the wig cap.

- Once your wig cap is secure, you can apply your wig. Position your wig where you want it to be, but peel back the front section.

- Use a wig adhesive or got2b Glued gel and apply a few dots along where you want to adhere the hairline of your wig. Using the tail end of a comb, smooth out the adhesive.

- Lay your wig's hairline on top of the adhesive and use a hairdryer to set. If you want, you can wrap a headscarf over the hairline while it dries, to keep it in place.

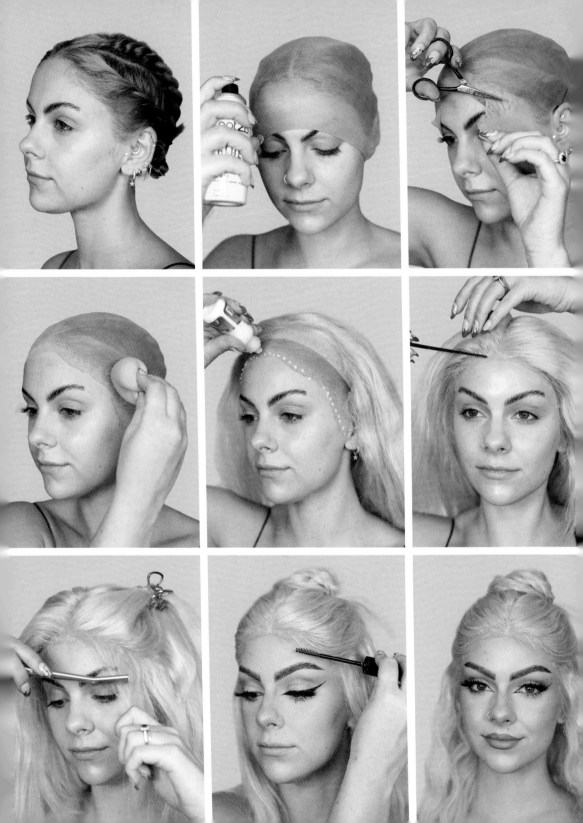

- If your wig didn't come with baby hairs, you can add them in if you wish. Use a tail comb to pull a small section of hair forwards, along the hairline. Trim them using a razor wand, spritz with freeze spray and comb them into your chosen position.

- Then you're ready to style your wig. Top tip if you want your parting to look more realistic: add a powder foundation along it, applied with an angled brow brush.

That's the most straightforward way you can install a wig, but you can definitely get away without doing a proper install if you're wearing a hat/bandana or headband, for example. Want to keep your wig installed for a while? They can last a few days to a few weeks if you look after your wig, be careful while washing it and sleep in a silk hair wrap.

REMOVING A WIG

When it comes to removing your wig, do not rip it off! Follow this easy guide to carefully removing it to take care of the wig and your skin.

- Tie the wig into a ponytail or clip back so you can clearly see the hairline.

- Soak a reusable pad or cloth in adhesive remover, then gently rub along the hairline to soften the glue. Cotton buds work well here too.

- When you can see the edge of the wig start to lift, carefully peel it away from your skin.

- Once the edges are peeled back you can remove the wig and wig cap.

- You will still have adhesive on your skin, so go back in with the remover.

- Then wet the hairline of your wig, as you will want to make sure this is clean for when you install the next time – you can use wig shampoo.

- If your wig needs washing (see overleaf), wash and air-dry it.

WASHING A WIG

Wigs should be washed, because if you don't wash them you will reduce the longevity of the hair. A wig is just like our own hair; if you're using styling products on it daily you can get product build-up or it can get dirty from the environment we're in. How often you wear your wig, how you style it and whether, for example, you work out in your wig, will determine how often you will need to wash it.

I'd recommend handwashing a 100% human hair wig under a shower head or tap with cool to warm water. When washing these wigs, look for gentle products that offer hydration – you want to avoid sulphates or anything that's going to strip the wig. With synthetic wigs, find a range tailored for these to make sure you're really caring for the hair.

And when it comes to drying the hair, air-drying on a wig stand is best, but make sure the hair is detangled first.

DYEING A WIG

Wigs can be expensive, but if you want to experiment with colour without the commitment to bleach, it's a great option. When I do this I always do so on a human-hair wig that's in a platinum-blonde shade, so I have a good base for vibrant colours.

There are a few ways in which you can dye a wig, and which method you pick depends on the style you've chosen. For example, if you want to dye just the money pieces, you can do this by securing the wig onto a canvas head and wig tripod stand, then apply the dye straight onto the hair. I do this for a lot of my wigs as I'm always applying multiple colours.

DYEING A WIG ON A WIG STAND

- Set up your wig stand and make sure the canvas head is secure.

- Protect the canvas head by wrapping it in cling film.

- Spray the lace of the wig with hairspray – this helps protect the lace cap from staining from the dye.

- Secure your human hair wig onto the canvas head and use pins to keep it in place.

- Brush through the wig, making sure all the strands are detangled.

- Wear gloves and have a dye brush and bowl ready to apply your chosen colour(s).

- Depending on how I'm dyeing the wig, I like to start from the underneath at the back and work my way to the front; this is how I would dye my own hair, beginning at the roots through to the ends of the hair.

- Once the dye is applied in your chosen style, leave it for 20 minutes minimum, then rinse under lukewarm water until the water runs clear.

- Use a microfibre hair towel to absorb any water from the wig, then air-dry it back on the wig stand – make sure to remove the cling film from the canvas head first.

However, if you're wanting your wig one shade, there is an easier and quicker method you can use.

DYEING A WIG IN WATER

- Fill a large basin or bowl with hot water and add in your semi-permanent hair colour. Make sure it's all mixed in – using a whisk will help.

- Spray the lace cap with hairspray to protect it from being coloured. The got2b Glued Blasting Freeze Spray is great for this.

- The more colour you add in, the more pigmented the hair will be. Do a little strand test before submerging the whole wig into the basin. When you're happy with the shade, submerge the whole wig into the coloured water. Make sure you wear gloves for this.

- While the wig is submerged, move the hair around, making sure it's getting evenly covered in the water. Leave submerged for 2–5 minutes.

- Repeat if the colour comes out patchy or not in the desired tone.

- Once you're happy, rinse under lukewarm water, use a microfibre hair towel to absorb any water from the wig, then air-dry back on top of a wig stand.

This technique also works well if you're wanting to tone a blonde wig to get rid of any brassiness. Instead of mixing hair colour with the hot water, you mix in purple shampoo.

Hairstyling

Experimenting with my hair doesn't stop with colour. From updos to waves to braids, I style my hair to express my personality or to complement the vibe of my outfit or the occasion.

Hair inspiration is one reason why people follow me on social media, specifically for my short-hair tutorials. Styling short hair can be tricky, a lot of people assume you can't do a lot with short locks, but you can style it just as much as someone with mid-long hair.

Here are some of my favourite go-to hairstyles that look amazing on short bobbed hair to long hair. So the next time you're looking for inspiration for a day out or even a wedding, come back here as I've got you sorted.

Daytime

When it comes to styling daytime hair, most of the time we're looking for something quick to do. Maybe we don't even do our hair in the morning before work, or we grab a scrunchie and chuck it in a top knot. If you do find you have five minutes in the morning, it's all it takes to create a nice wearable day hairstyle, and I have a few ideas for you.

CURLS OR WAVES

If your hair is naturally straight and flat like mine, you'll probably love curling or adding a wave to your hair. It instantly gives hair volume and a different finish that's wearable for the day or even makes a great base to work from to create many hairstyles.

There are so many different techniques you can use to curl or wave your hair, which each give you a different result. But personally, my favourite, quickest and easiest way to do this is with heated straighteners. Straighteners are a multi-tool, so I would always say it's worth investing in a good pair over lots of different curling tongs or wavers as you can achieve so many looks with them.

CURLING WITH STRAIGHTENERS

- Prep your hair with heat-protect and curl-hold spray.

- Starting with the underneath, you're going to section the top part of your hair and secure with sectioning clips.

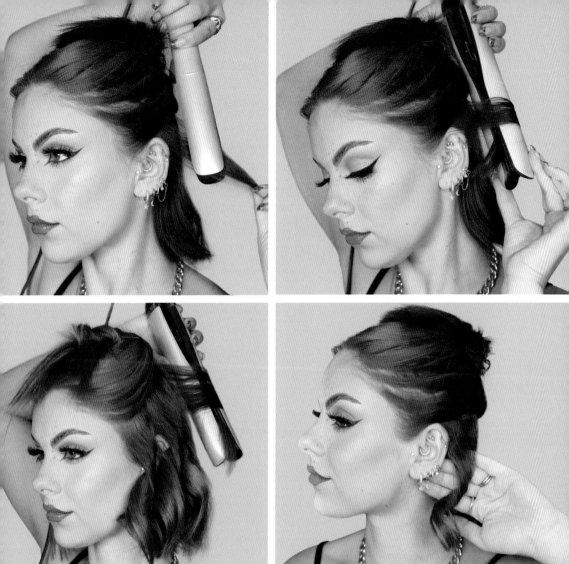
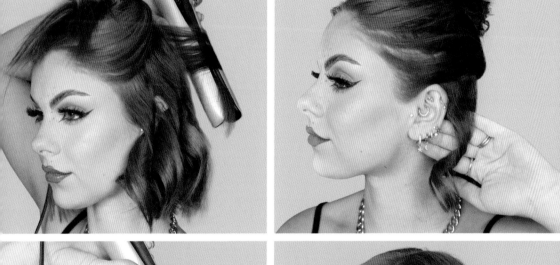
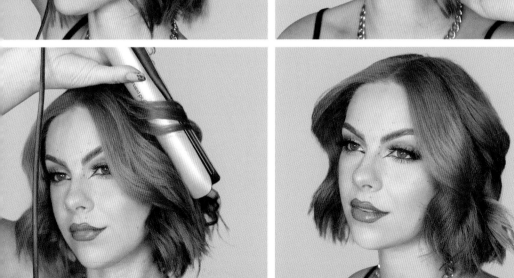

- Take your heated straighteners and take a small section of hair, about 2.5 centimetres wide, and place in between the styler at the root.

- Place the straighteners diagonally with the tip pointing downwards, then turn them one full rotation away from your face and while doing so glide down the length of your hair. You've created a curl! Keep doing this same technique, working in sections and dividing the hair as you go. Make sure you maintain the curling direction, so curl away from the face on both sides.

- Finally, use your fingers or wide-tooth comb to break up the curls and spritz a shine spray on top.

WAVING WITH STRAIGHTENERS

I have two amazing techniques to share with you on how to achieve a wave with straighteners. I love mixing these techniques together to add texture to the hair, but they also look great on their own.

S-wave

- Prep your hair with heat-protect and curl-hold spray.

- Section your hair as you would when curling. Starting with the underneath, divide the top section out of the way, securing with sectioning clips.

- Take your small section of hair and place in between your straighteners, holding your styler at a slight diagonal, next to your hair. Instead of gliding the straighteners down the hair, clamp the hair instead, gently.

- While clamping the hair, hold the section of hair below the straighteners and push it gently upwards to create a natural S bend. It can be tricky to master this method, but use the straighteners clamped on the hair to help you. Do this the whole way down the length of the hair and repeat all over. Try switching up the direction you start the S bend each time you do a section.

- Finish with shine spray and hairspray.

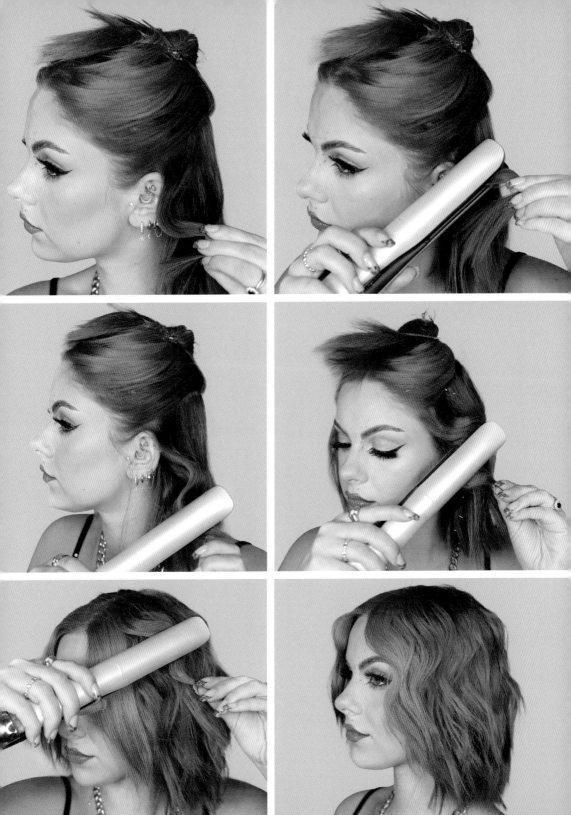

Beach wave

- Prep your hair with heat-protect and curl-hold spray.

- Section your hair, starting with the underneath, then divide the top section out of the way.

- Take a small section of hair and place it in between the straighteners and clamp down, keeping your styler horizontal.

- Pull the straightener upwards, holding that horizontal angle – this will give your hair lift at the root.

- The next part is all in the wrist action. Twist your wrist over and pull down, which will create a curve in the hair. Do this about 5 centimetres down the hair, then twist your wrist back on itself, which will change the angle of the straightener, pull down again about 5 centimetres to create another curve in the hair but opposite to the first one. Repeat this down the length of your hair. Twist your wrist to change the angle of the straightener, pull down, twist your wrist again, pull down. Always maintain the straightener horizontal to the hair, as this will create a tight wave.

- Working in sections, repeat over the whole hair and finish by combing through with a wide-tooth comb and a spritz of shine spray and hairspray.

If you prefer styling your hair through blow-drying, which I tend to do around 70% of the time, I'd recommend investing in a blow-dry brush, either the BaByliss Big Hair if you're wanting something affordable, or if it's within your budget the Dyson Airwrap is a great investment. The BaByliss Big Hair is great at achieving a big, bouncy, blow out, is easy to use and it even offers a design specifically for short hair as well as long. The Dyson Airwrap uses less heat compared to a heated styling iron, which in turn is much better for your hair. Styling through blow-drying will achieve great volume and I find it even makes my hair look visibly thicker and full. With the Airwrap you can achieve so many styles, from curls, to sleek and straight, to bouncy with flicked ends.

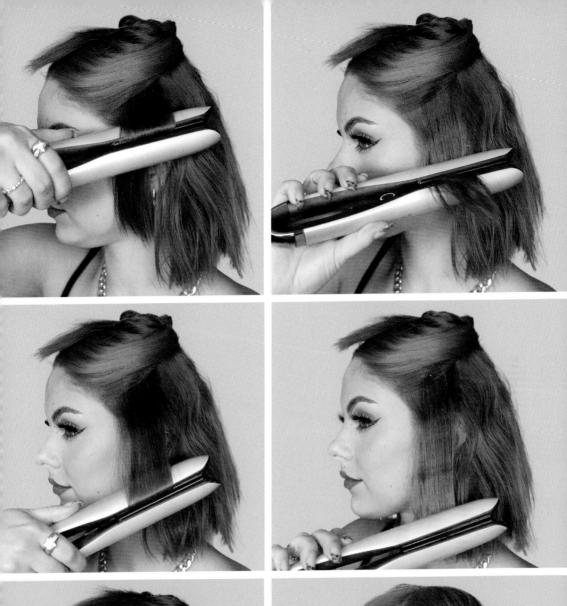

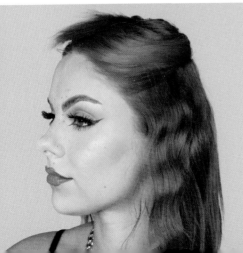

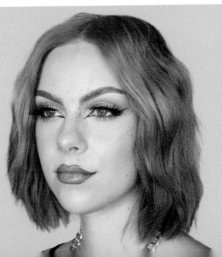

HALF-UP PIGTAILS

Half-up pigtails is a great everyday style. It works on most hair lengths and is simple to achieve, but it is also a great hairstyle to build from and make your own.

- Using a tail comb, part your hair down the centre, then divide a section on either side of the centre parting that will become your pigtails. There are two ways to do this: take a section from your ear to the back centre of your parting, or take a section from the tail end of your brow to the back centre of your parting. If you have bangs you can keep these out or include them in the pigtails.

- If all of your hair will go into the pigtail you don't necessarily need any hair products here, but if you are looking for a sleek look, use a hair gel to comb your pigtails into place.

- Secure your pigtails with a hair elastic.

It's as simple as that! The fun part is choosing what sort of pigtails you're wanting to achieve. You could curl or wave your hair before creating your half-up pigtails to add volume and texture to the overall look. Or if you're wanting a sleeker 'do, use straighteners to smooth your pigtails and create a flick at the ends.

If you kept your bangs out, you could comb to the side and add some hair clip accessories, even hide your hair elastics by wrapping hair around the pigtails or add colourful scrunchies that match your outfit.

That's what I love about styling hair. Once you've mastered a basic hairstyle step by step, you can add your own personality to the look.

FRONT BRAIDS

A favourite day look of mine, which works a treat if you're trying to grow out your fringe, is braiding the front sections of your hair.

- Style your hair with a curl or wave – I find this works better with volume at the back of the hair.

- Part your hair down the centre, then divide it into two sections, either side of the parting. Using a tail comb, start from about 5 centimetres back from the front of your hair and part from the centre parting to behind your ear. Using sectioning clips, clip the back of your hair out of the way.

- A braid milk, sheen or pomade, offers a little bit of grip that helps with braiding. Apply this product on the two sections of hair at the front.

- Then take three small strands of hair at the top of one section, where the parting is, and create a Dutch braid. Start off with a regular three-strand braid but cross the strands under the middle instead of over – so cross the right strand under the middle, then bring the left strand under the middle.

- Continue this method, but before crossing the left and right strands under, add a small section of hair to the strand. Do this down the whole section until you reach just past the ear.

- Secure with a hair elastic, tuck the end of the braid behind the ear and secure into place with a bobby pin. As an option you can pull on the edges of the braid to loosen slightly.

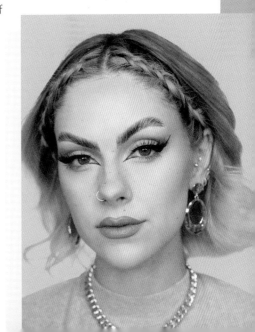

- Repeat the Dutch braid on the second section of hair, on the other side of the centre parting.

- Once secured behind the ear with a bobby pin, you can release the back hair you sectioned out of the way with sectioning clips.

- Spritz with shine spray and hairspray.

HALF-UP, HALF-DOWN CRISS-CROSS

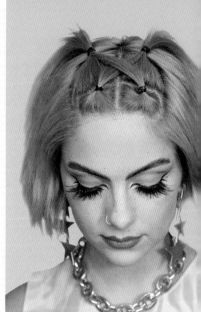

One of my favourites that's become rather popular on TikTok is a half-up half-down look where you create a criss-cross design using four sections of hair. This is another one of those hairstyles that you can build from. You could replicate this on smaller sections of hair, all the way along your hairline, as another look that would be great for a festival.

- Style your hair straight, curly or wavy.

- Part your hair down the centre, then part either side of the centre, about 5 centimetres wide. You should end up with two sections, starting from the front of your hair and going back towards your crown. Use sectioning clips to keep these separated and clip back the rest of your hair so it's out of the way.

- You're then going to split both of those top sections into two and secure with a hair elastic to end up with four small ponytails.

- Take the front left section and use a hair elastic to tie it to the back right section, then take the front right section, cross over the front left section and use a hair elastic to tie to the back left section. You will see you've created a criss-cross design.

- Remove any sectioning clips and spritz with shine spray and hairspray.

Evening

When it comes to the evening I always think glam and sleek. Something for a date, a night out or an evening with friends. You'll probably be in your best dress and you'll want a hairstyle to match. Here are four sleek hairdos to try the next time you're planning an evening out.

SLICK UPDO

Slicked-back hair into an updo oozes glam. It could be into a high ponytail, a low bun or even a Y2K spikey bun. You can slick all your hair back, slick it back with a centre parting or even a side parting to create an ultra-sleek, polished look. Obviously if your hair is longer than bob length, you will be able to properly twist the hair and wrap it into a bun, but this technique is great for short hair.

- Part your hair down the centre using a tail comb and spritz with water, then comb through with a hair gel. (I like to use the ECO Style Olive Oil Styling Gel – it's affordable, has great benefits for the hair and has a great hold.)

- Then comb the hair back so it's positioned about 5–7 centimetres from the crown and secure with a hair elastic. Spritz a strong-hold hairspray all over and pat down any flyaways.

- Coat the ponytail with a little hair gel and then twist the hair, fold it in half upwards so it creates a loop bun shape, and secure with another hair elastic.

- I like to leave the ends of my hair out so they're poking upwards then spritz these with hairspray into the position I want. This look is the ultimate Y2K vibe.

- Secure with hair clips any short hairs that haven't quite made it into the ponytail.

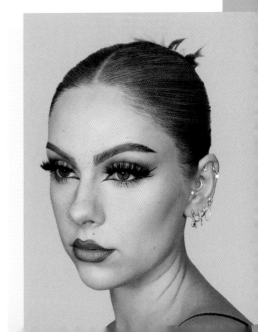

HALF-UP, HALF-DOWN SIDE PARTING

Another glam evening hairstyle is a simple half-up, half-down look, but with a sleek side parting. This works just as well on short hair as it does on long. This style also looks great with a high ponytail, if your hair is long.

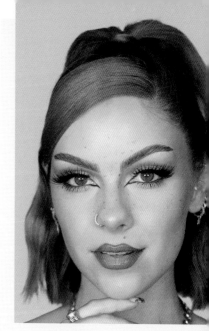

- Style your hair with a curl, wave or flicks on the ends. I find these three styles work well with this hairdo.

- Using a comb, section a semicircle at the front and centre of your hair. This will be the side fringe that you will secure later. Use a section clip to set it aside.

- Taking your comb again, divide the rest of your hair into two, creating a half-up, half-down ponytail. Section from your ears to the crown of your head. Use hair gel to slick this ponytail back and secure with a hair elastic.

- Take a small section of hair from within that ponytail and wrap it around, covering the hair elastic. Secure with a bobby pin, or if your hair is long enough you can take a topsy tail and use that to poke the hair you've wrapped around the ponytail, through it to keep it neat and secure.

- When you're happy with your half-up ponytail, take the section for your side parting and comb through with hair gel. Pick a side on which you want the hair to lie and comb downwards towards the ear, and if you can, tuck the hair over the ear.

- Use a bobby pin or hair clip to secure the side parting behind the ear. To make sure the clips are hidden, lay the back of the hair over the top.

- Spritz the hair with hairspray to finish.

WET LOOK

Another sleek and chic hairstyle is the wet look. This is literally where the hair is combed back and looks wet – it's that iconic red-carpet do. It's edgy, it's glam and when paired with a smoky eye can look sensational.

- Wash your hair and dry it with a microfibre hair towel so it's half dry.

- Mix in your palm a dollop of strong-hold hair gel and a dollop of styling cream. The cream will add moisture and eliminate frizz.

- Apply this mixture to your hair, running it from root to tip if you have short hair; for medium to long hair focus on root to mid lengths.

- Use a fine-tooth comb to smooth down roots and baby hairs and a wide-tooth comb to slick back the rest. Keep combing through until you achieve the slick wet look you desire.

- Once you're happy, spritz with a glossy shine spray all over.

- Mist your hair with strong-hold hairspray to lock in place.

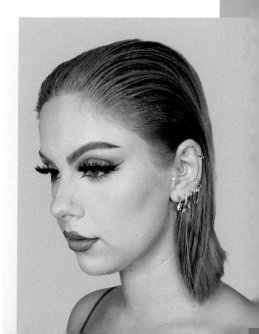

CURLY BUN AND FRINGE

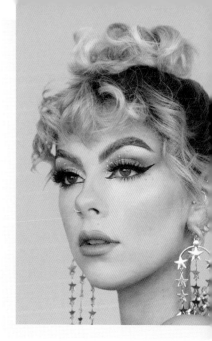

A not-so-slick updo that I love for an evening out is a high bun with volume from corkscrew curls and the addition of a faux fringe. It's another favourite look of mine, and when paired with glam eye makeup, this looks chic for a night out.

- If your hair is short, section a small semicircle of hair at the front and centre and clip aside. If your hair is long, go straight to step 2.

- Spritz your hair with water and comb it into a high ponytail, so it sits on top of your crown. You can add a small bit of styling cream or hair gel here depending on what sort of hold and finish you want.

- If your hair is short, you might want to use hair clips to secure any stray hairs into the high ponytail, or leave some out so that you can curl them.

- Spray the ponytail and fringe with heat-protect spray.

- Taking a corkscrew curling iron, curl the hair within the ponytail and the fringe section you clipped aside (if you have short hair). If you have any loose hair around the nape of the neck, you can also curl this too.

- Once the hair is curled, pull apart with your fingers to break up the tight corkscrew curls.

- If you have long hair, pull some of the curls forward over your forehead to create a faux fringe. Secure these in place using bobby pins.

- For those with short hair, the curls should already be a good length to act as a fringe, if not, you can pull the curls upwards, position them and use bobby pins to secure.

- Then use bobby pins to secure the curls in the high ponytail in place, so it creates a messy bun shape.

- Once you're happy with the position of the fringe and bun, spray strong-hold hairspray to keep the look locked in place.

Festival

When I create festival I looks, it isn't just the makeup that I get creative with, it's also the hair. I often get asked about these looks, so I'm going to fill you in on some useful tips, so you too can achieve some fabulous, colourful festival hairstyles.

BRAIDING HAIR

Firstly, let's talk about braiding hair, as this is a look I often use. I mainly buy my braiding hair on Amazon, and it comes in a variety of colours – it's synthetic and made from Kanekalon. When I'm planning my festival outfits, I will always opt for a colour that complements my overall look and colour palette.

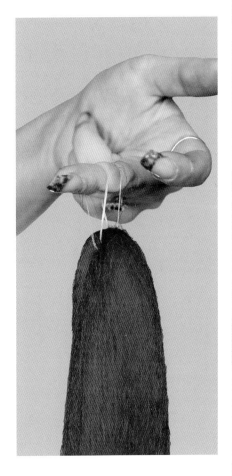

Braiding hair comes folded in half, with an elastic band tying it together in the centre. I utilise this and replace the elastic band with a hair band or hair elastic and make a loop with the hair band that can be tied around a ponytail or bun on my own hair. If you feel the braiding hair is too thick, you can carefully split it into two and add a hair elastic loop around each section.

Braiding hair can be tricky to work with, so I highly recommended investing in a conditioning braid spray like the Mane 'n' Tail Braid Sheen to make it more manageable.

Braiding hair is a way of adding colour, especially if your hair isn't dyed and you want a temporary pop of colour. Here are three other cute ways you can incorporate braids into your festival hairstyles.

BUBBLE BRAIDS

Bubble braids is a look I love for a festival, where you use lots of hair bands, evenly spaced apart down the length of a ponytail and the hair is slightly pulled out in between the bands to create a 'bubble' look.

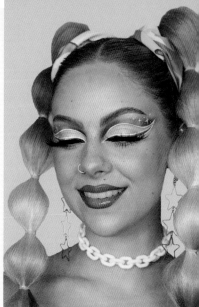

Using a gradient colour of braiding hair works well for this. Bubble braids are super easy to style and once you've mastered the technique, you can come up with so many different versions. You'll need a lot of hair elastics for this. Pick coloured ones to match your outfit.

- Part your hair down the centre from the front, down to the nape of the neck, using a tail comb. You'll need a mirror to check you've parted the hair evenly the whole way and once you're happy, use sectioning clips to keep it split.

- Using hair gel, comb your hair into two pigtails at your desired height. If I'm wearing a hat, I position my bubble braids low, if I'm wearing a crown I position them high. Secure with a hair band.

- If your hair is long, go to step 4. If your hair is short like mine, tie the pigtails into small buns and secure with a hair elastic.

- Taking your braiding hair, tie the loop around your pigtails (long hair) or buns (short hair. You're then going to start the bubble braid. If your hair is long, add it within the braiding hair and bubble braid the whole length. If your hair is short, cover the buns you've created with the braiding hair so that the first 'bubble' hides them.

- Start at the top of each pigtail and tie elastics down the length of the ponytail, keeping a consistent distance between them. After each section, pull gently on either side of the hair to create the 'bubble' shape. Repeat until you've created 'bubbles' down the whole length of the hair.

- To make it look neater where you applied the braiding hair, tie a scrunchie around the top of each pigtail.Once you're confident at creating bubble braids, try adding another set of pigtails to the hair and having four bubble braids – or even six! Why not jazz up your bubble braids with accessories like flower or butterfly clips, or rhinestone spiral twists?

MINI BRAIDS

If you're more into the boho festival style, wearing mini braids is a cute, easy look.

- Style your hair straight, with a curl or a wave. If you're camping and don't have access to electricity but want to achieve a wave or curl, you could opt for either sleeping in French plaits or wrapping your hair around a sock or dressing-gown tie, which will create a wave or curl when taken out the next day. I try to be strategic with my festival hair looks and tend to start the weekend with my hair down and by the final day it's in a fun updo to hide the greasiness!

- Create a centre parting, then take a small section of hair, pop some hair pomade onto your fingers and create a three-strand braid. Secure with a small hair elastic.

- Repeat this a few times on either side of the centre parting, creating mini braids over the top section of your hair.

- Finish off by accessorising with either adding beads at the end of each mini braid, or even by sticking rhinestones along the length of the braid.

This hairstyle works well on bob length to long hair.

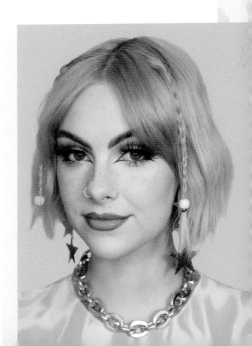

BRAIDED PIGTAILS

Instead of bubble braid pigtails, I love a simple three-strand braid using coloured braiding hair.

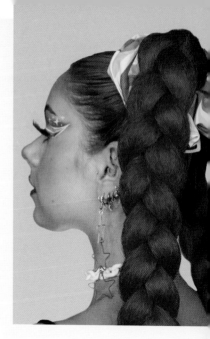

- Part your hair down the centre from the front, down to the nape of the neck using a tail comb. You'll need a mirror to check you've parted the hair evenly the whole way. Once you're happy, use sectioning clips to keep the hair split.

- Using hair gel, comb your hair into two pigtails at your desired height. If I'm wearing a hat, I position my braids low, if I'm wearing a crown, I position my braids high. Secure with a hair band.

- If your hair is long, go to step 5. If your hair is short, wrap your pigtails into small buns and secure with a hair elastic.

- Before attaching the braiding hair to your small buns, hang it on a door handle or something so you can plait the hair into a simple three-strand braid. Spritz the braiding hair with a conditioning braid spray to help manage the hair, then secure it with a hair elastic once you reach the tips.

- If your hair is long you won't need to pre-braid the braiding hair before attaching as you can include your long hair within it. Simply attach the braiding hair around your pigtails with the looped hairband, spritz the hair with a conditioning braid spray and split the pigtail into three before creating the simple three-strand braid.

- If you've pre-braided the hair, all you'll need to do is attach the loop over the small buns you've styled, lay the braid over the bun and use bobby pins to secure it onto the bun. Use a large scrunchie to neaten where you've attached the braiding hair at the top, so it discreetly hides the small buns.

It's as simple as that! And once you have your braided pigtails, the ideas are endless. You could have pigtails that have a few bubble braids and three-strand braids within them, or add chains or rhinestone trim, pom poms, fringing – anything goes with festival fashion. Personally, I think nothing is ever too much!

SPACE BUNS

Space buns is a classic festival hairstyle that works well on all hair lengths and types. I love that you can make space buns your own and that they're so easy to do. Space buns are essentially two buns high up on your head; you can work them into a half-up, half-down look or pull all your hair into them.

- For styling all of your hair into space buns, part your hair down the middle, from the front of your hairline to the nape of your neck. Use a tail comb and a mirror to achieve a precise parting. Use sectioning clips to keep the two sides separate.

- For half-up, half-down space buns, part your hair down the middle from the front of your hairline to the crown. Use sectioning clips to keep the bottom part of your hair aside.

- Depending on if you want a softer finish or not, you can either use hair gel or opt for no product to pull the hair into two high pigtails. Secure with a hair elastic.

- When creating the buns, there are many ways you can do this, it all depends on the finish you want to achieve. You could use hair doughnuts if you want a sleek finish, or for a messy finish twist the hair and wrap it around, not worrying if any loose bits poke out. Or you could three-strand braid the pigtails then wrap that around to create buns. Secure with a hair elastic and bobby pins to keep the buns in place.

- Use hairspray to spritz the buns and either flatten any flyaways for a sleeker look or pull little hairs out to add to the messy bun look.

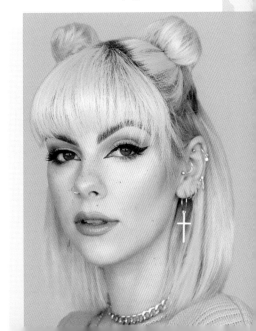

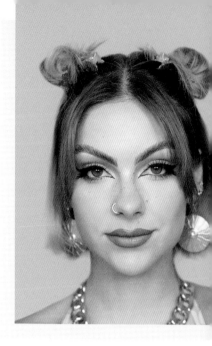

Space buns are quick and easy, and it's a hairstyle you can make your own with a few extras. There are so many cute ways you can add to your space buns look to complement your festival outfit:

- Add Dutch braids into the space buns: either at the front of your hair or from the nape of your neck upwards.

- Keep your bangs out of the look.

- Add accessories to your space buns, like little flower or butterfly clips or even spiral twists.

- Finish with colourful scrunchies or pom-pom hair ties.

- If your hair is long, add two mini braids at the front of your hair to pair with the space buns.

- Add glitter down the parting and use hair gel to adhere loose glitter to your hair.

Occasion

Special occasions always call for eye-catching hairstyles. Whether you're saying I do, going to prom with your date or have a big birthday planned, you'll want to look your best. I've got four versatile hairstyle ideas to share with you that will work for all your special occasions.

PEARL UPDO

Adding pearls into an updo instantly adds elegance and glam. There are many ways you can incorporate pearl accessories into your hairstyles, with bobby pins, headbands or even through embellishment. A chic and elegant up do that would make the most beautiful hairstyle for a bride or turn heads at your birthday party.

- Part your hair down the centre. Comb hair gel through your hair and pull it back into a low ponytail. Use a fine-tooth comb to achieve a smooth finish to the hair.

- Spray your hair with strong-hold hairspray.

- Taking a hair doughnut, place this over the ponytail. Cover the doughnut with your hair, then pop a hair elastic over the top of the hair, covering the doughnut. Tuck any excess hair under the base of the doughnut or wrap it around the bun.

- Secure the doughnut and hair into place using bobby pins.

- Spray strong-hold hairspray over the bun to smooth any flyaways.

- Adhere flatbacked craft pearls evenly over the hair using eyelash glue.

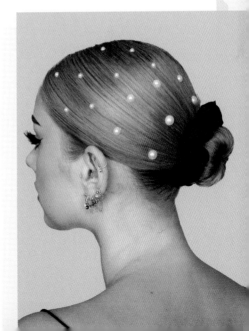

SIDE PARTING WITH CLIPS

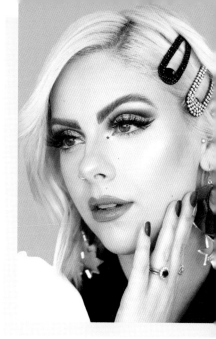

Voluptuous curls with a side parting gives me all the glam feels. Changing your parting can dramatically switch up your look and it makes the perfect hair for an occasion when accessorised with embellished clips.

- Ideally with freshly washed hair that's towel-dried, spray heat-protect and curl spray, then pick which side you want your side parting and use a hairdryer to tame the hair in the direction you'd like.

- Divide your hair so you can start with the underneath section. If you want volume and bounce, use something like the Dyson Airwrap or a round blow-dry brush. You can add volume at the root and curl while you blow-dry your hair from damp to dry.

- If you prefer styling your hair from dry, use a curling iron or straighteners to create waves or curls. You want to lift the hair at the root to create volume and curl the lengths of your hair.

- Curl or wave your hair from the underneath, working your way to the top section. When you reach the top section where you've parted your hair to the side, you're going to curl the side that will tuck behind your ear 'towards' your face and the side where your hair swoops over to curl away from your face.

- Once your hair is curled, spritz hairspray all over to lock your style in place.

- Grab a fine-tooth comb and some styling cream and comb the hair next to the side parting behind your ear.

- Grab some embellished hair clips that complement your outfit – gold if you're wearing gold jewellery, silver if you're wearing silver – and slide these into the hair you've smoothed down.

- Add a final spritz of hairspray and shine spray to finish.

SIDE PARTING WITH BRAIDS

Another side-parting hairstyle that's elegant for an occasion is adding a few loose braids instead of using embellished hair clips. The key to this look is that the braids sit on top of the hair.

- Follow the same steps as the previous hairstyle to achieve a side parting look with voluptuous curls, but instead of securing the side behind your ear with clips, you're going to divide this part evenly into two, using sectioning clips to keep them separate, then pop some matte pomade onto your fingers.

- Taking the top section you're going to create a three-strand Dutch braid. When braiding, keep alongside the direction of the side parting. Take three strands – take the left strand under the centre, then the right under the centre and keep doing this, adding a small bit of hair into the left and right side each time. You will only need to repeat this a few times as the braid will start from the front of your hair and stop by the time it reaches the back. When you've done one braid, pull on the edges to loosen it.

- Lift the back curls and secure the braid with a bobby pin or clip underneath, then lay the hair over the top to hide it.

- Take the second section of hair and repeat, creating another loose braid, that will sit alongside the other. Secure underneath the back curls.

- Spray shine spray and hairspray to finish.

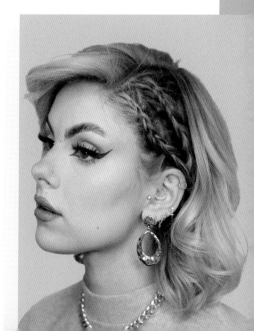

HALF-UP, HALF-DOWN TWIST

This classic hairstyle looks lush with long curls, however, it also works well on short hair and is beautiful for an occasion like a wedding or glam day event.

- Style your hair with a curl or wave.

- Take a section going from the middle of your brow towards the back of your hair, just under your crown. Tie this together loosely with a hair elastic. You don't want to tie too tightly to the scalp, leave a gap because you're going to twist it on itself. Place your finger in the centre, just above the hair elastic, making a hole, and push the ponytail through that hole and pull from the underneath. This creates a twist effect.

- Take a section of hair on either side of the first section and tie that together with a hair elastic, then twist that on itself too.

- Gently pull on the parts of the hair that have the twist effect. This will add volume to the twists, as well as texture.

- Once you're happy with how it's looking you can add an embellished clip just under the bottom twist or leave it as it is. Spritz with hairspray and shine spray to finish.

STYLING WITH ACCESSORIES

I'm a big fan of hair accessories, as they can instantly elevate your hairstyle, add in pops of colour and glamour, style your hair and keep it in place. I always find it's good to have a little pot of hair accessories to hand, because you never know when you'll need them.

CLAW CLIP

When in doubt, reach for your claw clip! It's a great go-to accessory for a daytime updo or even a slicked-back look for an evening out. Claw clips work for all occasions, and I love that they come in a variety of colours and designs. From a simple black design to tortoiseshell, metal or even a pastel flower shape.

There are a few ways you can wear a claw clip but the main go-to styles are putting all of your hair up or half of it. You can twist your hair into the claw clip, keeping it all secure, or you could leave the ends of your hair hanging out of the top for a more casual look. For a half updo, use a claw clip instead of a hair elastic to keep the hair in place at the back of your head. You can also use claw clips to secure space buns, or even add loose braids going into the claw clip updo. They're such a versatile hair accessory.

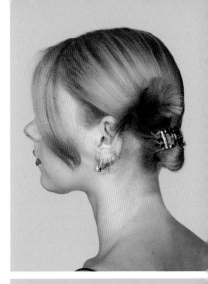

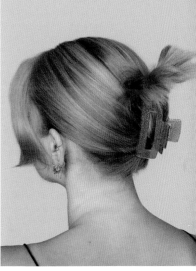

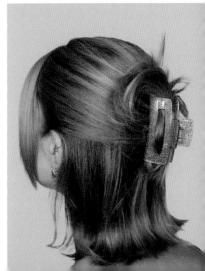

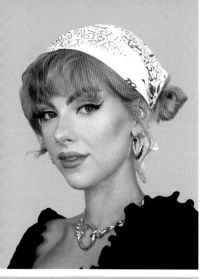

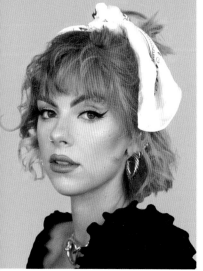

HEAD SCARF

Another favourite hair accessory is a head scarf, mainly because they can be worn in so many ways, but also because they can tie in with your outfit.

I love to wear a headscarf as a bandana; I fold it in half to create a triangle shape, then position it in the centre of my forehead and tie at the back of my hair. I find this way of wearing it edgy and either style my hair straight, flicked or curled with it.

I also like to tie a headscarf around a half-up, half-down bun to add a print or colour into my look that complements my outfit. If I've created a high bun, I wrap a headscarf instead of a scrunchie around it, or fold a headscarf into a long rectangle shape and tie it around my head, knotting it at the nape of my neck.

And finally, if I'm on holiday, I tie a headscarf into a 50s' pin-up style to protect my hair from the sun.

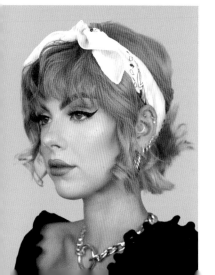

CLIPS

You should see how many hair clips I own – I have a box full! From neon to pastels, to star shapes to embellished ones, I think I have one in every colour! Hair clips work for all occasions – you can use them to pep up your hairstyles or to keep hair secure and in place.

I use hair clips for all sorts of looks, some of my favourites are:

Inspired by a hairstyle Rihanna wore in 2015, hair down and flicked out with hair grips along the front hairline.

Giving off Y2K vibes – I actually love that 90s/2000s hair trends have made a reappearance. Butterfly clips make any hairstyle look cute.

Tucking voluptuous curls behind my ears with embellished clip details at the front.

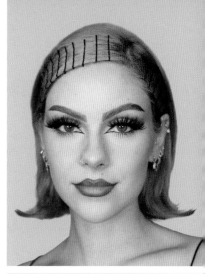

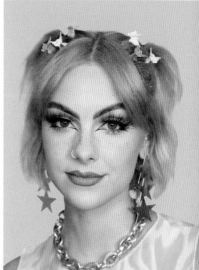

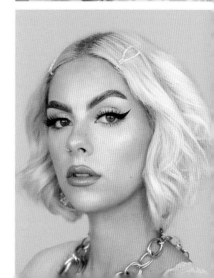

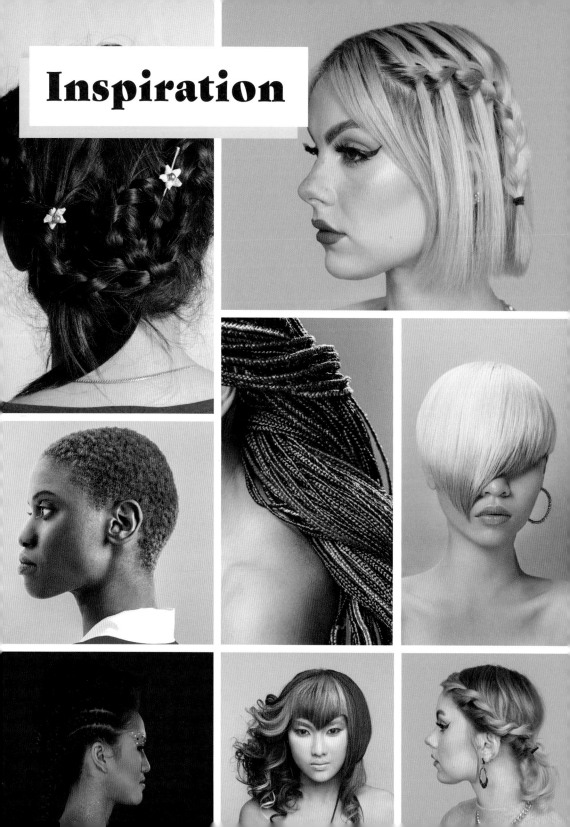

Inspiration

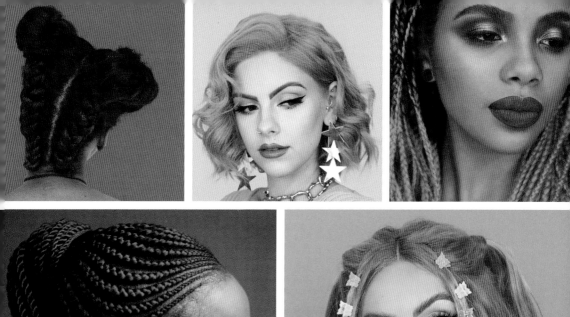
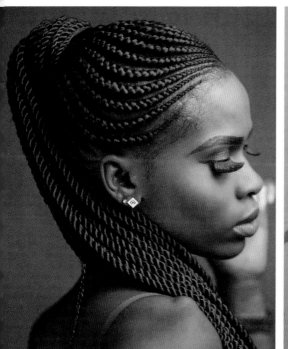
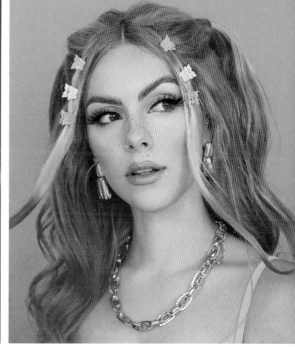
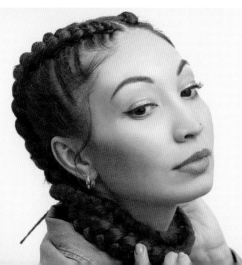
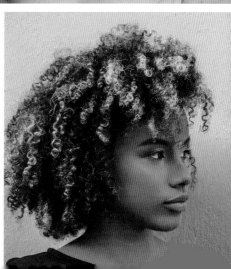

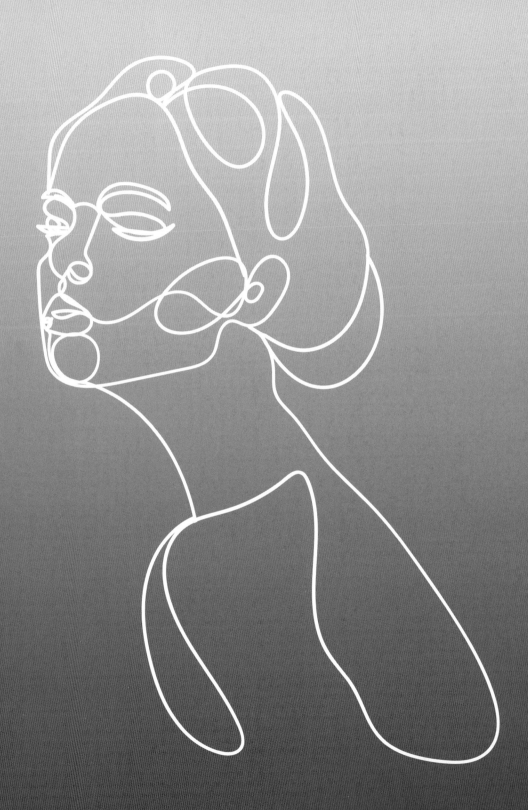

style

How to Have the Confidence to Wear Whatever You Want

I want to start off by talking about confidence. A comment I often see across my social media accounts is: 'I wish I had the confidence to wear that!' It always saddens me because nobody deserves to feel this way. We should all be able to dress and express ourselves however we choose. Most likely it's a body confidence issue or they're worried what people will think. Whatever the reason, the result is dressing so they 'fit in' and it's just such a shame.

I'm not going to pretend that I haven't had similar thoughts. Our minds can limit us, our inner voices can talk us down, but if you can overcome those negative thoughts and wear that outfit you love, I guarantee you will feel incredible for it! No matter how confident you are, it's natural for a negative thought to cross our minds.

I bet if you've followed me for a while, you've assumed I've never ever considered 'not' wearing an outfit, but I've put on an outfit and thought, maybe there's a little too much showing? But then I look at the outfit and I think no. I LOVE it, I love how I've styled it, I'm obsessed and I'm wearing it! And you know what? I've never once had a comment from someone saying 'oh you're showing a bit too much wearing that'. The comments I've had are 'You look amazing!', 'Your outfit, oh my god', 'Where did you get it?' and the recurring one... 'I wish I had the confidence to wear that'.

Among those amazingly kind comments people say to me about my outfits, I know there will be someone thinking the opposite. No matter what you wear, how you do your makeup or hair, someone will dislike it. We were never born into this world to all be alike. We are all so different and that goes with our likes and dislikes as well. Luckily, though, in my 30-plus years I've never had anyone say anything negative to my face. It is hard to not worry about what other people think, but we can't control other people's negative thoughts and reactions, but as I can't hear their thoughts, I just wear the outfit I want to wear.

I was reminded recently that while you're spending time worrying about what others think of you or the way you look, the fact is that the other person is probably not even thinking about you at all, because we each individually have a lot going on in our lives. Ok, someone might have a quick thought of 'I don't like that person's dress', but do you know what? I guarantee within minutes they've forgotten it and they're back to thinking 'what shall I cook for my dinner tonight?'.

I know it's a cliché, but after losing my dad young, life really is too short. You never know when your last day will be. So wear what you want to wear and don't think about anything else, other than how good that outfit makes you feel! And I'm sure if you ever sit there one day reflecting on past years, you won't have any regrets about any of those incredible outfits you wore. You'll be happy that you wore them!

'Don't be into trends/ Don't make fashion own you, but YOU DECIDE what YOU ARE, what YOU WANT to express by the way you dress and the way you live.'

GIANNI VERSACE

Our Bodies and The Fashion Industry

One thing that can affect the way we dress is our bodies and the way we see ourselves. A key contributor to low self-esteem is the fashion industry and the certain type of model that they will only represent. We interpret that as if we don't look like that, or have that figure, then we're not good enough, so we don't wear what we want to because we don't look like the model that advertised the outfit.

Fashion brands are slowly getting better at being inclusive and representing more 'real' women as they realise the effect it can have on a consumer. There are more and more brands every day starting to represent a range of shapes, sizes, ethnicities and disabilities. There is still a long, long way to go, but it's a positive change, which I think we can all agree has been needed for a while. It's hard enough still having magazine and celebrities being airbrushed and photoshopped.

One thing I love to see is the amount of content creators that now talk about body confidence and self-love. They play such an important role in changing how we view our bodies, by showing us what 'real' women look like. Social media doesn't have to be another place that makes us feel down about the way we look, it can be uplifting and relatable, you've just got to know where to look. A good place to start if you're needing a pick-me-up is searching the hashtag #bodypositvity on social media. Or if you're after finding body-confident creators, start with these amazing ladies: Alex Light, Sarah Nicole Landry, Ariella Nyssa, Megan Jayne Crabbe, Tiffany Ima and Nelly London.

Loving your body is easier said than done, and you're not alone in feeling low about the way you look. Changing the way you think and see yourself takes work but there are lots of different ways you can work on body confidence and self-love.

1. **Reflect** – ask yourself why you don't feel confident. Dig deep to understand what it is that's making you feel that way, and uncover your thoughts and beliefs. Changing your mindset is hard when you don't understand why you feel the way you feel.

2. **Be kind to yourself** – it's so easy to focus on the negatives and talk ourselves down. Don't lose sight of how much our bodies do for us. Practise gratitude and remember how remarkable our bodies are. We might have a few things we dislike about them, but why not instead focus on the bits we do like? That's a great place to start feeling confident – dressing to highlight the parts of your body you love.

3. **Become more self-aware** – something that has come as a result of having therapy and that has helped me tremendously in the way I think is the fact that I'm more aware of my negative thought patterns. And because I'm more aware of the negative thoughts and how they affect me, I can stop myself, change my mindset and let go of the negativity, then feel more positive and content. Try to become more aware when you next have a thought about your body.

4. **Stop comparing** – we were born to be different and unique. Comparing ourselves will only lead to a negative mindset.

5. **Surround yourself with people who uplift you** – you deserve to have people in your life who are positive about you and make you feel good about yourself. Don't ever let anyone put you down.

6. **Unfollow on social media** – we spend a lot of time on our phones, on social media. If someone isn't making you feel good about yourself – maybe you're struggling not to compare yourself to them – mute or unfollow them. Make your feed a safe place that uplifts you and leaves you feeling good when you come off the app.

7. **Accept you for who you are** – you don't need to change the way you look. You ARE beautiful the way you are. You ARE enough!

8. **But if you're really struggling with confidence and body image, please talk to a mental health professional** – they are there to help. Mind.org.uk and Samaritans.org.uk are good places to start.

Dressing for Your Shape

Personally, I believe anyone can dress however they choose, regardless of their shape. Dressing for your shape is a concept that's been around for years and it's something that feeds into this idea of 'looking slim'. Depending on your body shape you'll be told to avoid certain styles because they can be unflattering, or that you should wear a certain style of garment to draw attention away from another area of your body.

I think dressing for your shape is more of a personal preference to help ourselves feel good and comfortable, about trialling different cuts, colours, fabrics and prints to figure out what works for you and your aesthetic. Through years of experimenting with clothes, I do find myself drawn to certain shapes and styles, but I've never been fixated on dressing for my shape and looking into all the body types. I dress for me and to highlight a certain aspect of my body that I love. We all have bits that we like, so show them off! That's how your confidence can grow.

We can all wear whichever style of neckline, trouser or dress length that we want to. Don't avoid clothing because society is telling you to, because you never know, you could be missing out.

Personal Style

Style is how we choose to express ourselves, and one way we all do that is through how we dress. Our clothing can showcase our personalities, our hobbies, and even our mood. Some of us might choose to follow trends, but most of us will have our own personal style and aesthetic that has developed over the years. It's certainly not something that you can figure out overnight, but there are things you can consider while deciding on your own personal style.

1. **Look at your wardrobe:** pull out a few of your favourite pieces, do they have something in common? Why are they your favourite items?

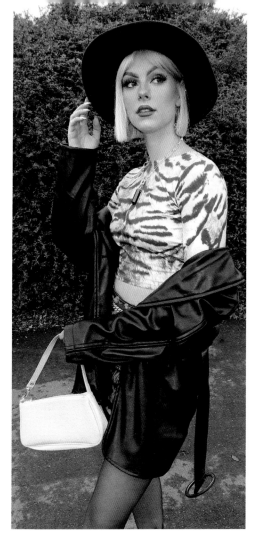

2. **Inspiration:** make a mood board, whether that's on Pinterest or Instagram, save outfits you're drawn to. You'll definitely notice a pattern emerging when you look at the overall images you've saved. Maybe it's that you love nude or all-black, or perhaps bold prints.

3. **Experiment:** how are you going to figure out your personal style if you haven't experimented with different looks? Take yourself down to the high street, get in the changing rooms and have a 'trying on' day.

4. **Focus on you and what makes you feel good:** who cares if it's not on trend, or if someone else doesn't like it. Remember, you're dressing for 'you', nobody else.

When it comes to your personal style, don't feel like you must fit into one box – you can like lots of different looks. Don't think you can't buy something because it's not your usual style. If you like it and it makes you feel good, wear it!

My personal style is a bit like that. I love a colourful wardrobe and clothes with a bit of an edge, but I also love to wear all black and look chic. We can have multiple styles, and we can choose to express ourselves differently depending on the occasion or day. And if your style changes? That's ok! As we go through different stages in our life, our tastes and aspirations change, we grow, and our style evolves with us.

How to Shop

Experimenting with our personal style and the way we dress doesn't come cheap. It also doesn't come without having an impact on the world. There's so much to think about when we shop – from the price, to the fabric, to the way the garment was manufactured, to the ethos of the brand you want to buy from and what they support. For some people those things won't matter, but for a lot of us we want to make sure we're making the right purchase, not only to make us feel good, but to meet any beliefs or opinions we might have.

I know when I shop I look out for certain things. I love supporting small brands, finding quirky statement pieces. I like to know if the brand is making a conscious effort to be as sustainable as they can be and that they're inclusive. On the odd occasion I stumble upon a piece on the high street I can't take my eyes off, the rest of my thoughts go out of the window because I'm hooked. However, if you know where to look and how to do the research you should be able to find something similar from a brand or shop that meets your values over buying fast fashion.

I'm not going to pretend that I never buy from fast-fashion brands – I do. Not all of us have the luxury of being able to afford the more sustainable option, as they tend to be higher priced. However, if you shop around and think before you buy, you'll realise there are a lot of other ways of shopping that can be a lot more cost-effective, and that can help the environment.

Second-hand is a great way of shopping. Ok, you might pick up some fast-fashion pieces, but at least the items aren't ending up in landfill and are being repurposed. Great places to look for second-hand clothing are charity shops, car boot sales, apps like Depop, Vinted, Facebook Marketplace, eBay and vintage shops. Second-hand shopping can be rewarding when you find an amazing bargain, however, it can often be frustrating when you don't find what you're looking for. You have to have patience with second-hand shopping; it might take you four or five visits to different charity shops before you find an item you are looking for, compared to visiting one huge fast-fashion shop on the high street. But it can also be thrilling, a fun day out or afternoon surfing the web with a cuppa, and it'll meet a lot more of your values.

Another way of being sustainable with your wardrobe is instead of buying a new dress every time you have an occasion, you rent one! Yes, there are rental apps for clothing – I don't know why it took so long for it to become a concept, as we can already rent a lot of things. Some shops like Selfridges in London, are even jumping on this clothing rental idea. You can rent a dress for a day, a week, however long you need it for. The perks are that you can wear something from a designer that you probably could never afford to buy for yourself and it's sustainable because you are avoiding adding another item to your wardrobe that you might only wear once if it's for a special occasion. The only negative would be that it can be costly, especially if the amount of days you want the dress for add up – for example, if you've had to rent a dress for an occasion abroad like a wedding. It's a great option, but not one that would be affordable for all.

Some people might not like the thought of second-hand clothing, and that's fine; you can still be sustainable while buying something brand new, or finding items that have been handmade or produced with a limited number of resources. This is how I shop a lot of the time, because these brands tend to be independent, crafted beautifully and produce pieces you can keep for years. Brands like this, I find, are worth investing in and once I'm done with the pieces – if I ever am – I donate them or sell them on. Sustainability doesn't just come into play when buying clothing, it's also a consideration when you have a wardrobe clear-out.

Let's talk about fabrics, as this is another way of being sustainable. I have to say I am impressed with more and more brands now selling garments made from recycled fabrics. It's hard to avoid buying fabrics like polyester, but if you can opt for a garment that's been produced from recycled fabrics, you'll be helping the planet by keeping plastic waste away from landfill and the ocean. If you want to be more conscious about the fabrics

'Being sustainable in the fashion industry is a challenge, and no fabric is truly environmentally impact free; but there are certain factors that will help. Small and slow fashion brands are good places to start, as they will use smaller quantities of often higher-quality fabrics. Plenty of brands use deadstock fabrics (which in truth are the most sustainable as they already exist) and will often create and sell garments until the fabric has run out, then move on to a new style. Although these brands often have a higher price point, the price can almost always be offset by the quality of garment and lessened impact on the environment.'

MIRANDA STANFORD, OWNER OF MONDAY'S CHILD LONDON

you buy, look out for organic hemp, cotton, linen, bamboo, vegan fabrics and wool (depending on how it's sourced).

How many times have you rummaged through your wardrobe and found a top you haven't worn in years? Or even one with the label still on it? I can hold my hands up and say that's been me before! I always think before I make a purchase now and ask myself, will I wear it often? Do I need another green top or bikini? One of the best things you can do is buy less, because most often we don't get round to wearing it all anyway. Instead, why not invest in timeless, high-quality pieces that you can keep and restyle each time you wear them. That's one reason why I love dressing myself, seeing how many ways I can style up a key wardrobe staple.

Let's talk about wardrobe staples, because these are always great to invest in. Garments like a pair of blue jeans, black jeans, jumpers, blazers, t-shirts – basic items that are so handy to have as part of your wardrobe. They work for most seasons, and you can mix and match them with statement pieces. Everyone's wardrobe staples will be different as we all have our own unique personal styles and garments we might prefer wearing over others, and different budgets, but here's a good guide to help you when you're next organising your closet.

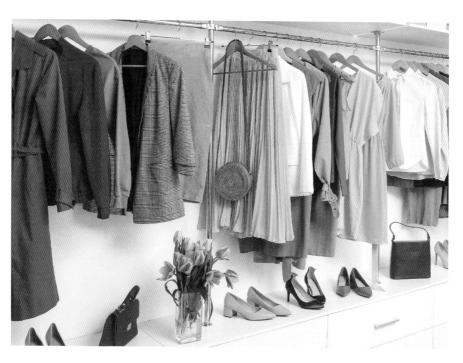

WARDROBE STAPLES

KNITWEAR
A knitted sweater or cardigan, whichever you prefer, is a great staple garment. Layer it in winter and wear it on cool evenings in summer. Looks great styled with jeans, skirts, leather trousers, even over a dress.

DENIM
Denim is always a great go-to. Denim jeans can be dressed up with heels and a top for an evening out or dressed down with a tee and sneakers for a more comfortable day look. I'm a trouser girl at heart, so a pair each of skinny, mom and straight leg jeans and I'm sorted.

WHITE BUTTON-UP SHIRT
Another great addition to your wardrobe. Pair it with a tailored look for something smart or wear unbuttoned over a summer dress. Maybe you want to utilise the collar and layer it under a knitted jumper or dress? A white shirt is such a versatile wardrobe piece.

LBD
You literally can never go wrong with a little black dress. It's classic, timeless and chic; you can dress it down for a day look and wear it with tights and boots, or go glam for an occasion and pair it with high heels. You can style many looks with an LBD just by switching up your accessories and shoes.

LEGGINGS
Wear them around the house, to the gym, for a comfortable day outfit or even with heels and a blazer for a night out. A pair of black leggings is definitely worth investing in.

LEATHER TROUSERS
Leather or faux-leather trousers are great for those occasions where you want to look stylish and chic – maybe you've got an interview, an event or dinner. These trousers can be mixed and matched with many different looks, from pairing with shirts to knitwear, or even a hoodie!

SNEAKERS

I live in sneakers! They're my go-to shoe for a day look, especially if I've planned on doing a lot of walking. A pair of white or black sneakers are a great staple.

DENIM OR LEATHER JACKET

Having a go-to denim or leather or faux-leather jacket is always handy to have as part of your wardrobe. Layer it up in the colder seasons or even take on holiday with you for those chilly summer evenings. It's an all-year-round garment you can wear for so many different occasions.

WHITE TEE

You can style a basic white t-shirt in so many ways. It can be glammed up or worn to the gym. You can use it to layer and wear under corsets, jumpers, even dresses or dungarees. Or you can wear it on its own and pair it with a blazer, bomber jacket or even cycling shorts.

BASIC TURTLENECK

More of an autumn and winter staple, but a turtleneck is great for layering. Wear it under knitwear or dresses, or even with trousers and a blazer. A turtleneck is chic and can add warmth to an outfit in the colder months. I have a white and a black basic turtleneck in my wardrobe and I always pull them out in the colder months.

BLAZER

I am a big blazer fan, especially an oversized one. I like the coolness it gives to my style. It can act as a jacket for an evening out, look smart for work or an interview, be layered in winter and even worn with jeans.

RIBBED TANK TOP

This can look chic worn under a blazer, or casual worn with a sweat set. Or pair it with fitted jeans, heels and a chunky chain for a cool outfit for a night out. I have a few ribbed tank tops in white, black and even block colours like green and orange, which pair well if I'm wearing a statement-print blazer or trouser.

BLACK SKIRT

You can never go wrong with a black skirt, of any length – mini, midi or maxi. You can work a black skirt into many looks and in winter still wear it, but paired with tights.

CAMI TOP

A little strappy cami top can be paired with trousers, a skirt, under a shirt or jacket. It's a basic that's wearable all year round.

SWEAT SET

Since the pandemic I think we've all got a sweat set in our wardrobe, but did you know they're a great staple, not just for around the house? A sweatshirt or hoodie paired with a blazer can look super chic in autumn and winter. Or even wearing a blazer over the top of the whole sweat set together, paired with boots, makes a great comfy outfit for a day of shopping. A sweat set is also a travel outfit go-to and I even take one to festivals with me when I'm glamping.

SLIP DRESS

A mini, midi or maxi slip dress is another all-season staple. It's the perfect lightweight dress for summer – a slip dress makes a great wedding guest dress – but it is also stylish for winter as you can experiment with layering: over a shirt, over knitwear, with a blazer. You can leave a slip dress loose or even add a belt and cinch it in at the waist for a different fit.

SHOES AND ACCESSORIES

Finally, let's not forget shoes and accessories. If you follow me, you'll know I love to style my outfits. It doesn't stop with clothes, I think about the jewellery, the bag, the shoes, the belt. I feel accessories are where you can really express your personality and inject your own style into your look. Your accessories can reveal a lot about you; you might be minimalist and keep it simple with no jewellery, or you might go bold with necklace layering, all the earrings and a bright bag.

Great shoe and accessory staples are:

- **Black and white handbag** – super-chic, and white goes with everything.

- **Black sunglasses** – sunglasses are a handbag necessity. Not only do they offer UV protection for your eyes, you can find a pair to suit your personal style.

- **Black heels** – you can't go wrong with a pair of black heels, they literally go with everything.

- **Black boots** – another staple shoe for your wardrobe. Black boots are great for spring, autumn and winter and if you're not a high-heel-sandal wearer, they're a great alternative if you prefer a boot style because you can get a heeled pair for your closet.

- **Sandals** – owning a comfortable pair that go with every outfit that you can chuck on every summer is key! There's no point in buying a new pair for every holiday you go on. If you've already got some that don't give you blisters, you're winning!

- **Hoop earrings** – a classic and chic earring style to wear that works for day-to-night looks.

- **Chain necklace** – from thin to chunky, adding a chain necklace completes the outfit. It adds personality, and jewellery can become such a keepsake item.

- **Black belt** – not only useful for holding your trousers up, a belt can break up a bold outfit, cinch your waist to highlight your shape or even keep a blazer secure so it doesn't flap open. A black belt is a great staple as it works with all colours.

Wardrobe staples never go out of style so it's always worth investing in quality pieces if you can, whether that's second-hand, vintage, or buying from a sustainable independent clothing brand.

Prints and Colour

You've got your staples sorted, but what about the rest of your wardrobe? Depending on your personal style you might want to add in colour, prints and patterns, or even monochrome clothing. When you open my closet, you're met with a lot of colour and prints. I have my basic items, but I'm constantly drawn to anything bold. I'm an outgoing, artistic and creative being and I think that really shows through the way I dress. I like to find statement, unique pieces that I can style differently each time I wear them.

I want to share how you can wear prints and colour and introduce both into your wardrobe in a way that's not too overwhelming. Then as your confidence grows, you can experiment more and more. Wouldn't it be amazing if you could just wear what you wanted when you wanted?! Obviously for some things there's a time and a place. I mean, I'd love to dress like I was going to a festival every day, but that's not realistic. One, because it takes me a few hours to get festival ready. Two, because it's not seasonal-proof, especially in the UK! And three, there's such an enjoyment in getting ready for a festival, if I did that every day, it just wouldn't be the same.

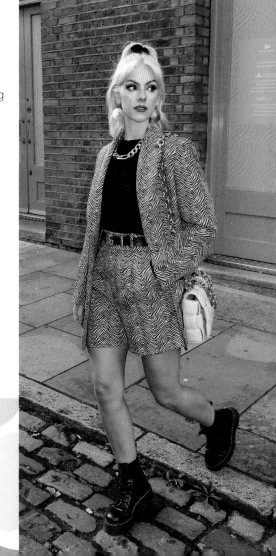

PRINTS

Wearing prints can be daunting, as there's a lot to choose from! Then there's figuring out which print goes with what. But hopefully with my top tips on how to wear them, it'll give you the confidence to try something new.

First let's look at what prints are most popular: gingham, stripes, animal prints, plaid, florals, polka dots, geometrics, paisley, checks and houndstooth. All of these are timeless, so they are great to have in your wardrobe, as they never go out of style.

Whenever I wear a bold print, I always look into the colours that are a part of it and tie those in with the rest of my look. For example, if I was to wear a check blazer with a colour palette of white, pink, blue, green and yellow – when it came to styling the rest of my outfit I can create many combinations by focusing on those shades. I could pair it with a white cami top and pink trousers, or a yellow top and blue denim jeans. If you stick to the colours within the prints, your outfit is guaranteed to work.

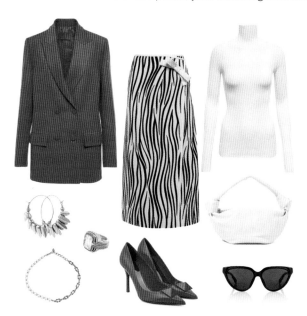

Clashing prints isn't something I personally like to do, because my style is all about 'matching'. However, it does work and it can be bold, fun and stylish. When experimenting with mixing prints, start off with patterns with the same colour combinations, such as monochrome black and white prints in stripes and polka dots, or mix a pink and red floral print with a pink and red stripe. Then when you're

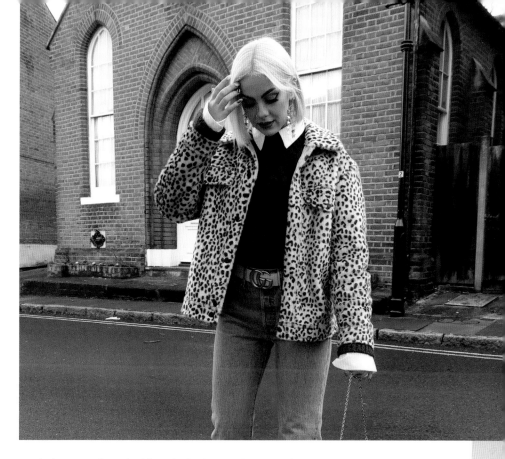

ready for something bolder, clash a leopard print with a plaid. You're probably thinking, wow, that sounds like a lot, but tie a plain item into the look as well, such as a white blazer or black belt, and it'll break it up. Another way of wearing prints is to choose and pair patterns of different sizes, like a small floral print with a large check print.

My favourite way of wearing a print is as part of a co-ord, like a jacket and skirt or trouser set. So I wear one statement print then break it up with a top that ties into the colour palette from the pattern of the print. Co-ords are a great wardrobe addition because of the many combinations of outfits you can create. You don't have to always wear the pieces together, you can wear them as separates too.

If in doubt, go for a black-and-white zebra print paired with a bright colour. Probably one of my favourite prints to wear, it looks so stylish paired with neon green, hot pink or blue. To be honest, zebra print works with every colour and animal prints are timeless.

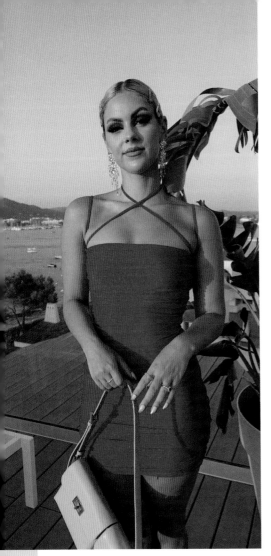

COLOUR

Colour might not be to everyone's personal taste, you might be one of those people that's 'all-black everything', and that's absolutely ok. Some people find it safer sticking to blacks, whites and neutrals, which looks super-chic if your style is more minimalist. 'I don't know what colour suits me' can be a fairly common thought for a lot of us. When it comes to fashion, though, there really aren't any rules. Yes, there are colours that can enhance your natural complexion, the exact same way makeup does. But as with makeup, anything goes. It might be a good place to start wearing colours that will naturally suit your skin tone, but in all honesty, if you love the colour and feel confident wearing it, it won't matter. Wearing bright colours is known to lift our moods, after all. And for me, it really does! It gives me a boost.

Colours for skin tone:
Cool skin tone – try bright greens, deep purples, pinks, blues, and silver
Neutral skin tone – try white, red, jade green and mid blues
Warm skin tone – try greens, browns, reds, oranges and golds

If you want to add colour into your wardrobe, start small with statement-coloured accessories: bags, sunglasses, shoes, hats, a hair scarf or scrunchie and jewellery. You don't have to wear something bold to add colour to your looks.

Another great place to start is with pastels; they're not so in your face and work well in spring and summer. You don't have to introduce colour all at once, start with a single item of clothing like a coloured top, and pair it with jeans and a white jacket. You also don't have to stick to block colours, so try a print with subtle colours and when you feel confident, go bolder with the print and hue.

I love complementing colour combinations, all-one-colour looks and coloured prints. I've always been a wearer of colour, which has meant over the years I've discovered what my favourite combinations are, and they've become a part of my personal style. The saying goes: 'blue and green should never be seen', but my god whoever said that got it so wrong. Those two colours together work so well and it's one of my go-tos. Along with pink and green, purple and green, pink and orange and pink and purple.

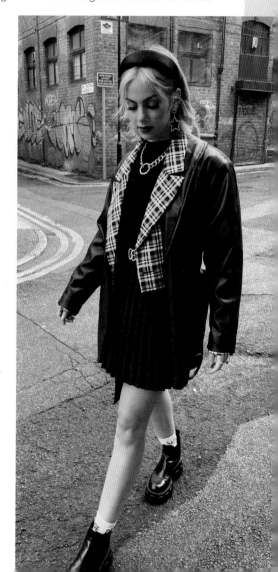

And when I'm not mixing colours, I love creating monochrome looks by picking one bright colour and wearing it from head to toe. I also like to mix same-colour fabrics, so pairing green faux leather with green satin, for example. If you can't find the same shade of the one colour you want to wear, don't worry, combining a dark and light shade of the same colour in an outfit looks flawless.

I'm forgetting I've always got coloured hair, and that comes into play whenever I'm styling my outfits. I find most of the time it doesn't matter what colour my hair is, it always works and never looks out of place or too much. As long as you're confident, it'll show, and it'll suit you.

Layering

Sometimes it can feel tricky to add your own personal touches to your winter outfits because of all the layering that's needed to wrap up warm. It's all about experimenting, trying out different colour combinations, mixing fabrics and patterns. Here are a few of my go-to ways that I love to layer in winter without losing my own sense of style.

LAYERING A DRESS

You can transition your summer looks into winter using layering. Got a favourite summer dress you love? Depending on the neckline why not pop a long-sleeve turtleneck top underneath, high-denier tights, socks and boots and finish with a lined faux-fur coat.

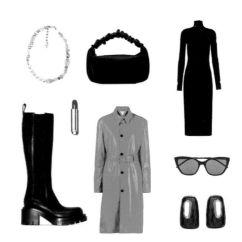

SWEATER VESTS

A knit sweater is, I'm sure, everyone's winter go-to. But I sometimes find it can be a bit boring just shoving on a jumper every day throughout the colder months. That's why I adore sweater vests. You can layer a long-sleeve basic top under a white shirt then pop a cosy knit sweater vest over the top. Paired with jeans, sneakers or boots and a long trench coat, you'll look stylish and, most importantly, be warm.

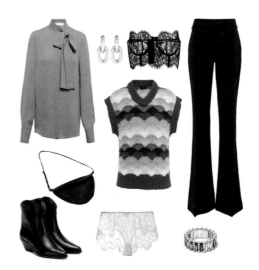

TURTLENECKS

I've mentioned that a turtleneck is a great wardrobe staple and it really is for the colder months. For me, it's also my number one layering item. I wear one under t-shirts, shirts, dresses, sweaters and blazers. Having a basic turtleneck is great, but it's also good to have a statement colour or print-style turtleneck. It can really elevate your outfit and you can use the print or colours within its design to tie in with the rest of your look.

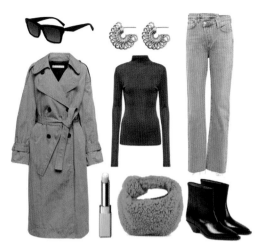

DOUBLE COAT

Yes, I love layering a coat over a jacket or blazer. For those days where it's just a little too chilly, those extra layers are needed. For the outer layer, I tend to opt for a length that's longer than the jacket underneath. A great layering combination is a belted blazer with a long faux-fur coat over the top, or another favourite is a teddy bomber jacket with a hood paired with a faux or leather jacket over the top.

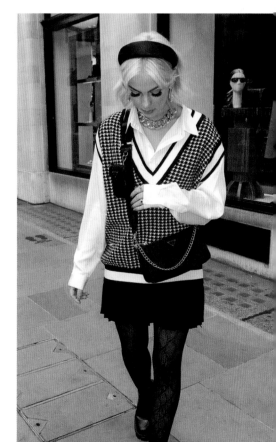

Accessorising

You've got your staples and you've added in some prints and colour. When I'm getting dressed my favourite part is styling the look and adding any finishing details. This, for me, comes down to the accessories – it's the ultimate way to add personal style.

You're probably wondering how you can read someone's personal style through their accessories. Think of it this way, if I were to see someone wearing coloured jewellery, I'd get the sense they'd be a bit eccentric. But if I saw someone wearing a simple thin necklace and hoop earrings, I'd think they're chic and minimalist.

It doesn't take long to pop on a pair of earrings or use a belt to cinch in your waist to highlight your shape. These finishing touches can really elevate your outfit, so I'd recommend having a few accessories on hand whenever you're getting ready 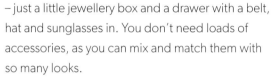 – just a little jewellery box and a drawer with a belt, hat and sunglasses in. You don't need loads of accessories, as you can mix and match them with so many looks.

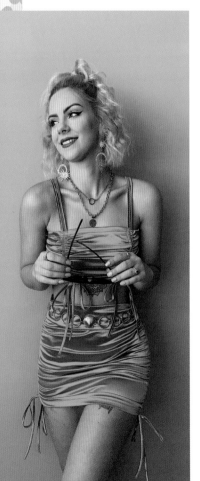

When I'm putting outfits together, I always accessorise with jewellery. I feel naked without it! I pick either silver, gold or a colour – whichever complements the overall colour palette of my outfit – then I opt for big earrings, a chunky chain necklace and rings. They're my go-to, then in summer I might wear a bracelet, belly chain or anklet as well. Jewellery is another area where I receive a lot of compliments and questions. I do have eleven ear piercings – so that's probably why!

On the topic of jewellery, it can be a lot to think about; but you don't need to wear every item you own. If I'm wearing a halterneck top, for example, I avoid necklaces because I've already got detailing around my neck from the top. Same with bracelets, if I'm wearing long sleeves, then I tend to not bother with bracelets as they're usually never seen.

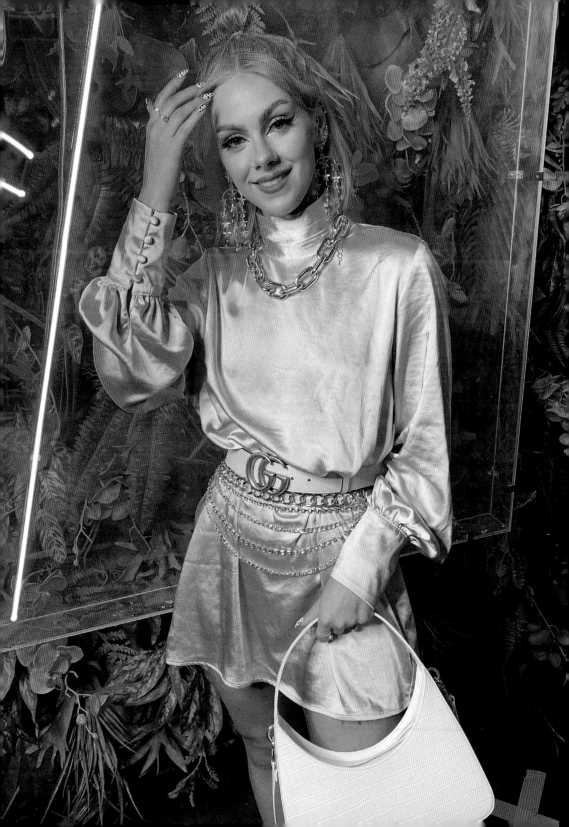

Occasions

I don't know about you but getting dressed for an occasion brings me joy. It's different to your everyday wear, so occasions are where you can really elevate your looks, get creative, stand out from the crowd and dress yourself up to think 'I look incredible in this'.

If you follow me on social media, you'll know I have a bold, quirky style, I'm always drawn to unique pieces, colour, prints and anything matching. I'm going to share my favourite occasions with you and how you too can use these to express yourselves and dress so you feel and look your best.

PARTYWEAR

From black tie to outdoor events, parties can be daunting to buy for when there are so many different dress codes. So I thought I'd make things easier for you and give you the lowdown on various party dress codes and a bit of a guide on looks that suit. I've been there, after receiving an invite, thinking 'where do I even start to look?' or 'what counts as a black-tie dress?'. So, the next time you receive an invite, pop back to this guide for inspiration.

BLACK TIE

This style of party is formal – think gowns and tuxedos. You don't have to wear black; colours are also an option. Dresses should ideally be mid- to floor-length in metallic, sequin, satin, lace or beaded fabrics. Something elegant but glam. If you're not into dresses, a smart, tailored suit works just as well. When it comes to accessories, pearls and diamond drop earrings pair well, and for an evening bag a detailed or statement clutch is perfect.

COCKTAIL

A cocktail party or event allows for more choice. You can have a bit more fun and go bold and make a statement – try a puff-sleeve mini dress or a gradient sequin dress with a slit, or you could grab your wardrobe staple LBD (little black dress). It doesn't have to all be about dresses, you can switch it up and wear a jumpsuit, playsuit, suit or separates. For trousers you can go for a wide leg sleek trouser in something like satin or keep them more tailored. You can wear colour, prints, or keep it chic and wear black. With accessories you can make a statement with a unique pair of heels or oversized earrings and big jewels.

FESTIVE

The festive party season is all about sequins, velvet, metallics, satins and festive colours – something that's going to help you sparkle the night away. You can have fun with festive wear and when in doubt, wear sequins! What I love most about partywear is that once you've found your perfect party dress or top that you feel amazing in, you can re-wear it time and time again. Partywear is timeless! Your LBD can make an appearance for a festive party; why not pair it with diamanté jewellery for that added sparkle. You can even pull out your best jeans and pair them with a sequin top and high heels or boots. Or why not try a blazer dress – smart, but dressy and glam.

With accessories, get creative and go all out. Statement jewellery pieces, oversized dangly earrings or even chain belts. With shoes, you don't need to stick to heels, you could wear platform or over-the-knee boots or even flat brogues. Match your bag to the colour of your outfit or go for a statement sparkly clutch.

Wear what makes you feel fabulous!

SMART CASUAL

Smart casual might be a dress code on a party invite but it's also a great option if you've got a dinner date, work party or day event. This dress code always throws me off, but I've managed to pull it off on many occasions purely by thinking of it as 'dressing up' a casual look. And by dressing up I mean, pop on some heels or heeled boots, statement jewellery, slick my hair back into an updo and add a smart handbag or clutch. You can wear jeans for a smart-casual look if you pair it with a nice top, something satin or sequin, maybe even a corset. Or if it's a day party wear a summery cotton dress but instead of flat sandals or sneakers, wear heels and jazz up your makeup and hair. You can style a smart casual outfit easily by literally mixing casual pieces (jeans, cardigan, floaty skirt) with more dressy pieces (tailored blazer, sparkly top, tailored trousers).

OUTDOOR

Dressing for an outdoor party compared to an indoor can be slightly different. Think garden, beach and waterfront locations. If a party is outside, most of the time these are during the summer months as, ideally, the hosts are hoping their guests are going to be able to dance in the sunshine. With that in mind, think summery prints, bright colours, pastels and white or light fabrics. You could wear a floaty maxi dress, ruffle mini dress or a co-ord set. Crochet, broderie anglaise, lace and satin are all great fabrics to look for. Look out for cutout, statement straps, backless and slit details, they work great for an outdoor party. Remember, if it's outdoors the weather could be hot, but it could also be chilly or rain. It's always good to check the weather a week before so you can be prepared if you need to take a little wrap or cardigan.

Accessory-wise, anything that you feel complements your outfit will work. Coloured jewellery can tie into your look, especially if you're wearing all white, and those little details can make your outfit pop. With shoes you can keep them to flat sandals or heels, it'll depend whether you'll be partying on grass or sand. Finish off with a little summery bag to complete the look.

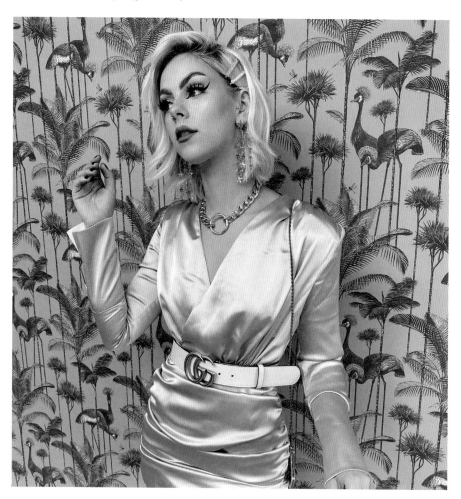

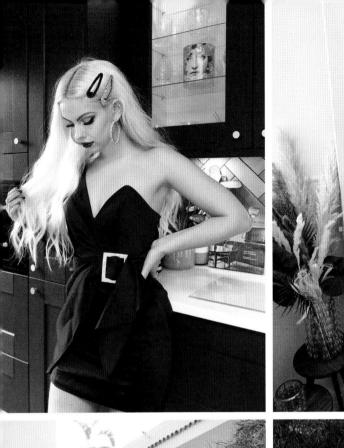
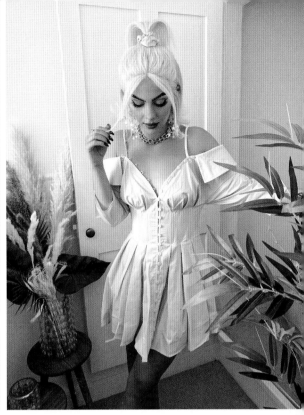
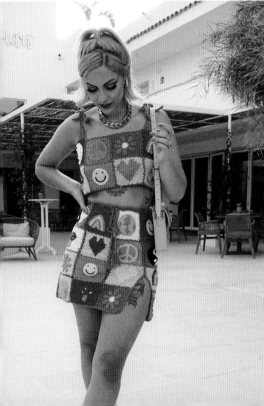
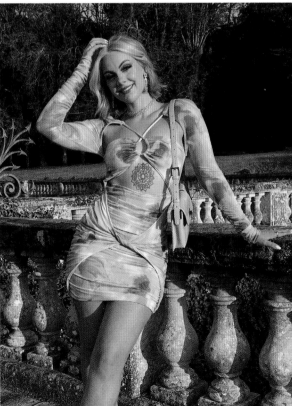

WEDDINGS

Don't you just love a wedding? A day filled with love, family, friends and just good vibes. Everyone will have a wedding to attend at some point in their life and when that happens you might be faced with 'what do I wear?', especially if it's your first one – they get easier after that! It's not just guests thinking about what to wear, though, the biggest decision for their outfit is most definitely for the bride(s) and/or groom(s). When two people come together to say their vows to each other it's a special and memorable moment and you both want to feel and look your ultimate best.

I got married back in 2018 wearing the biggest Cinderella dress and blue hair – yup! BLUE HAIR! Weddings don't have to be stereotypically traditional; they can be whatever you make them. The day, after all, is about you and your partner. If you're a Bride-to-be or a Groom-to-be, stay true to yourself. Don't try to 'fit' into the traditional wedding attire, unless you want to, of course. I actually never pictured myself wearing a white dress. I thought I would have chosen a colour or black. I mean, I had all of those saved on my Pinterest board, but when it came down to it, I thought, this is my only opportunity to wear a big white dress, so I'm going to wear it. My hair was my colour, it ended up being my something blue. Overall, with my whole look you could see my personality and personal style shine through. I am obsessed with sparkles and glitter so my dress was covered in them! And for shoes … If you google 'wedding heels', ivory or white satin, strappy heels will pop up. I went for the complete opposite and found these eccentric platform boots with a sun, stars, cloud and flowers on. They were a statement and to me they sort of represented the wedding day in a boot, and the main colour was blue so they matched my hair – of course! Then there was my wedding jacket, which is becoming a thing to have now, with either your new surname on if you change your name or 'just married'. Mine was a blue sequin jacket with my new surname in a sequin heart on the back, again, very 'me'. I didn't really stick to any wedding rules when it came to my big day and you don't have to either. Just remember, it's yours and your partner's day, ignore all opinions and do you! Trust me, you won't regret it!

In some ways, weddings are all the same, but in others they can be very different. This will depend on the religion of the couple, for one thing. When attending a typical formal wedding as a guest there are a few unwritten rules. The obvious being don't wear white, ever! It's kind of obvious but let the bride(s) have their moment. Even if the bride wears black or a colour, always assume they're going to wear white.

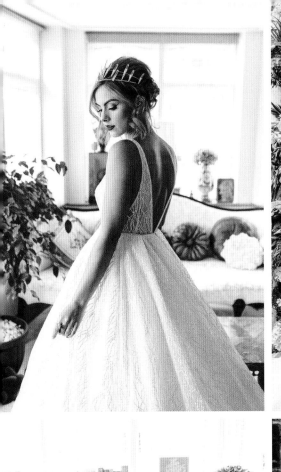
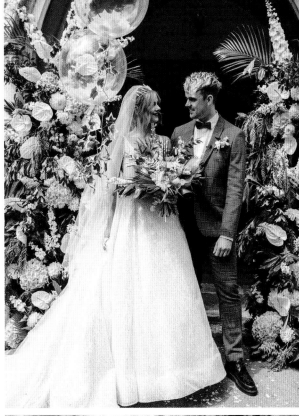
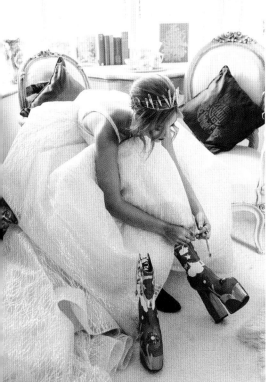
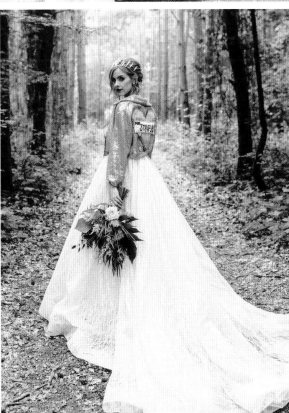

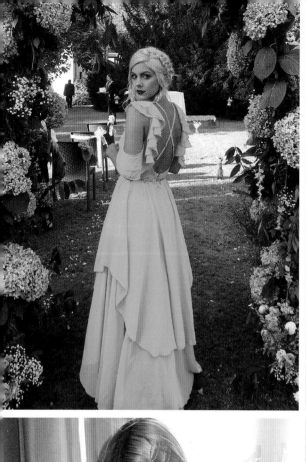
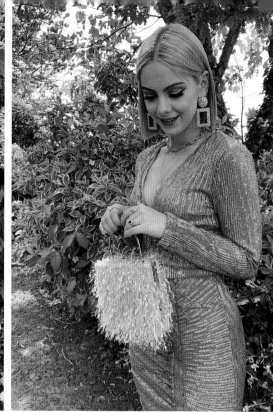
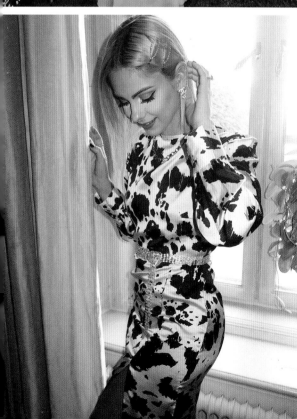
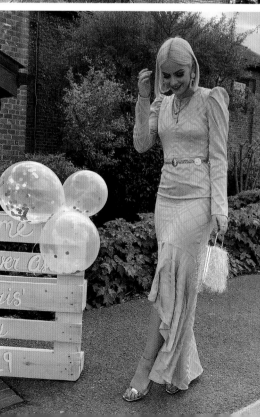

If you can find out what colours the bridal party are wearing, it's always a good question to ask the bride as it's best to try to avoid those shades. Opting for a print can sometimes help you avoid this, as bridal parties often wear solid colours. Try not to go too casual, obviously avoid jeans and t-shirts, but if you feel more comfortable in casual fabrics try to opt for something a little fitted, for example, dress up a cotton jumpsuit with a cropped tailored blazer and heels. Want to wear trousers? Go for something tailored and pair with a matching blazer or a statement blouse. Think about your shoulders, if the ceremony is taking place in a church setting, for example, be respectful and if needed add a shawl or cardigan to your look, which you can then remove later for the reception. Don't forget your neckline either; remember, weddings are family occasions with guests of all ages, and sometimes religious. That's not to rule out a plunge neckline, just consider if it's too much.

Avoid overdressing and outdoing the couple: you don't need to wear a gown or dress with a train, so don't risk drawing attention away from the bride(s) or groom(s). And finally consider the wedding's aesthetic, location and season. Is the wedding on a field in a stretch tent or is it abroad on a beach? Maybe a grand manor house or chateau? This will help when considering your outfit, as will the season. If it's hot, you will want lighter fabrics with short sleeves, maybe something loose-fitting. Then with colours and prints you can opt for brights, florals and pastels. Whereas for a winter wedding, you might go for deep jewel-toned colours, velvets and satins, maybe something with a long sleeve. Overall, weddings tend to be fairly formal, often you'll find dress codes have been set, but you'll always be safe wearing smart casual to evening wear if a dress code hasn't been mentioned. But if you're ever in doubt, ask the couple that are getting wed.

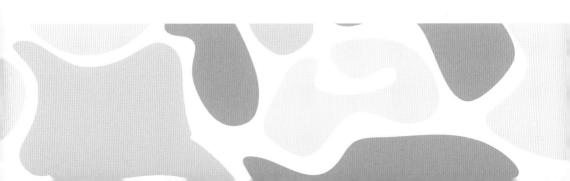

SUMMER HOLIDAY

My summer holiday wardrobe always excites me. I can't tell you know nice it is to put on a dress or skirt and top and not to have to worry about covering up your outfit for warmth. Don't get me wrong, I love layering in winter, but it is nice to just put on a dress and accessories and be out the door without thinking, 'what jacket will go with this?'.

Everyone's summer holiday wardrobe will be unique to their personal style. I love bright colours, neons and prints and am always drawn to co-ord sets, however, it's always good to have some staples on hand when you're packing for your trip. After all, you're confined to taking a suitcase and there's only so much you can fit in.

A few great holiday staples are:

- **Day-to-night dress** – a floaty maxi style is perfect for this – something lightweight and loose-fitting. Or even a crochet midi dress that you could wear over a bikini during the day but pop over a slip dress at night.

- **Wide leg trousers** – great for wearing with a bikini top during the day and dressing up with a blouse or top in the evening. Wide leg trousers are so versatile; look for lightweight fabrics like linen or jersey that'll keep you cool in the heat.

- **Basic tops** – plain neutrals or coloured tops are handy to pack as you can mix and match them to create multiple outfits.

- **Mini/midi skirt** – whichever length you prefer, take a few skirts with you on a summer holiday. These can be used to create outfit combinations paired with your basic tops.

- **Oversized shirt** – useful to throw over a swimsuit or bikini as a cover up, but you could also wear it with a belt and sandals to create an evening look.

- **Denim** – shorts or mini skirt, without a doubt I always pop a pair in my suitcase. Again, great for throwing on over a swimsuit, but can also be paired with a nice top for an evening outfit.

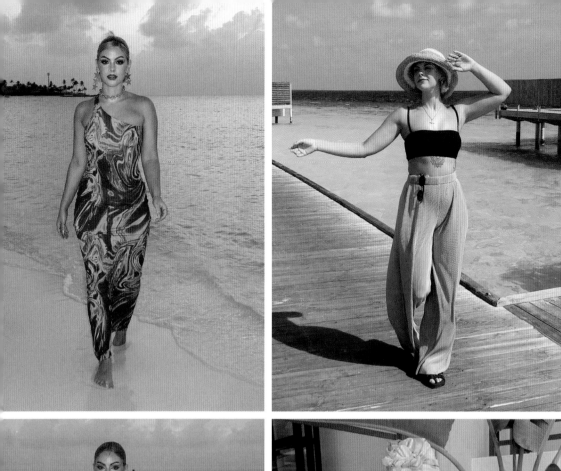
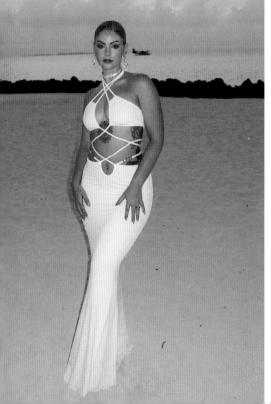
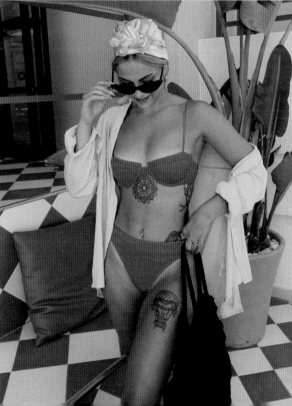

- **Beach cover up** – you don't need a different beach cover up every day of your holiday. I like opting for a shirt and short linen set as they're comfy, loose-fitting and lightweight. With a set you can mix and match the top and bottoms with other items you've bought with you, like the shirt with denim shorts or wide leg trousers.

- **Swimwear** – pretty obvious for a holiday, but finding a swimsuit or bikini you feel comfortable in is key to making you feel good while you're away. You could keep it simple with an all-black or all-white swimsuit or bikini or find one to suit your personal style with a print. There are so many different styles of swimsuit on the market, it's definitely worth trying a few to find what you feel comfortable and confident in.

- **Sandals** – the key here is comfort. There's nothing worse than blisters from your sandals while you're away. A pair of flats that are easy to slip on are so useful for the beach or days out. Then if you want to wear heels, switch things up for your evening looks with a pair of heeled sandals. Choose a neutral colour like nude, black or white so they complement your whole holiday wardrobe.

- **Sunhat** – to keep your hair and face protected from the sun. Also very handy if you're a book reader while you sunbathe.

- **Beach bag** – crochet, straw or canvas, find a bag that's a good-enough size to fit all of your essentials in: beach towel, sun cream, snacks, water, book.

- **Sunglasses** – another obvious one, but there's nothing worse than forgetting your sunglasses when you go on holiday. I like to take a few affordable pairs in different colours and designs to mix and match with outfits, plus it's always handy in case I lose a pair!

Staples are great, especially when mixing and matching and throwing over swimwear; but no doubt you will also pack some statement pieces for evenings out. From playsuits to jumpsuits, co-ords and dresses. Wear outfits you're going to feel comfortable and confident in.

FESTIVAL

My absolute favourite occasion to dress up for is a festival. Part of the experience for me is my outfit. It's the one place that's judgement-free, everyone is there for a good time, to let their hair down, and you can be creative or as out there as you want with the way you dress. You'll see trends each year at festivals but personal style plays a big part in choosing your outfit. For the most part, anything goes.

I plan my festival looks well in advance; mainly because this is when I like to support small, independent brands who often handmake the clothing so the lead times can be a month or so. If you've followed me for some time, you will have noticed I theme my festival looks, as this helps me overall with planning my hair, makeup and accessories.

The key to my festival looks is 'matching'. Firstly, I find the outfit that acts as the core of the look. Then whichever colours or prints it has, I find accessories to match. With accessories I like to go overboard, because why not?! I look at earrings, rings, necklaces, belts, gloves, tights, socks, hats or headpieces. If I were to do a star-themed look, all my accessories would feature stars; for a heart look, the accessories would have hearts all over. Through matching, the whole outfit ties together seamlessly.

When it comes to accessories, sometimes if I have time I will DIY a hat or headpiece. This happens if I have a vision of my festival look in my head and I can't find the perfect accessory as my finishing touch. A plain headband or Western-style hat with a glue gun, rhinestones, fringing and embellishment and you're off.

Let's talk about footwear. I'm not going to lie, I always struggle with shoes because I feel like I manage to style amazing outfits, but with shoes I let down my looks. The key to festival footwear is comfort over style. You're going to be on your feet for a few days, dancing and racking up those steps, so you'll want shoes you know you'll feel great in. Sneakers are the best option, I like platform ones to give my outfits a bit of an edge or, if you prefer, boots are also a great alternative. I have a pair of white cowboy boots that are so versatile and will work with the majority of my festival outfits; they're comfy and they're chic. And as much as I hate wellies, they're a backup option you've got to consider, especially if the weather is going to be wet. With loads of people walking on a wet field, it'll get very muddy, very quickly.

Regarding wet weather, it's always good to think about outerwear for a festival. I tend to opt for a poncho that's small and can fit in my bag, then I style a fun jacket over my outfit; something usually with sequins. Festivals tend to have lockers available, which are totally worth spending the money on.

The level of how 'festival-y' I take my outfits to is dependent on the festival I'm attending. For example, I've been to Coachella a few times and the vibe is quite boho, day glam, whereas something like Electric Daisy Carnival, which is during the night, is ravewear, so it's bright colours, light-up garments and accessories. It's worth considering the vibe when planning your looks; however, I tend to be one of the most dressed at festivals and it never bothers me because I feel amazing in my outfit. If you love festival fashion, go for it, just like I do. And if you don't and prefer a more comfortable, typical daywear look, that's totally fine as well.

I often get asked where I shop for my festival clothing. It's one of my most-searched blog posts on my website, I've included my favourites in my shopping guide at the end of this book.

If the way I dress up for festivals doesn't quite match your personal style, there are so many other outfit styles might appeal to you:

- **Head to toe in denim** – the great thing about this aesthetic is it fits every type of festival from country to rock.

- **Sheer dresses** – cool and sexy, a festival is the perfect excuse to try a sheer dress, layered over a bikini or swimwear. You can find sheer dresses in short to maxi length, in bright or neutral colours or a pattern.

- **Crochet** – a crochet matching set with a combination of a skirt, top and hat or even a crochet dress paired with cowboy boots makes a cute, comfy festival look.

- **Matching sets** – something colourful, sequinned or with fringing, a matching set is always a good go-to for a festival. All it needs is a personal touch with your favourite outerwear, shoes, jewellery and bag.

- **Floaty dress** – if your style is more boho, a floaty maxi dress with boots could be the perfect festival look for you.

- **Baggy jeans/trousers** – go for basic blue jeans, sneakers and a bikini or statement top or find some jazzy printed baggy trousers.

When it comes to festival fashion, be yourself, anything goes and have fun with your looks. But don't forget – comfort is key!

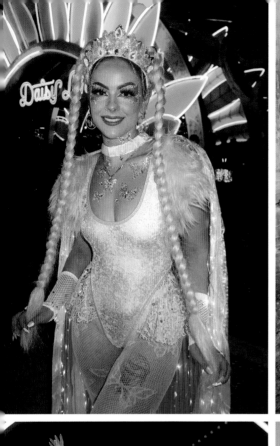
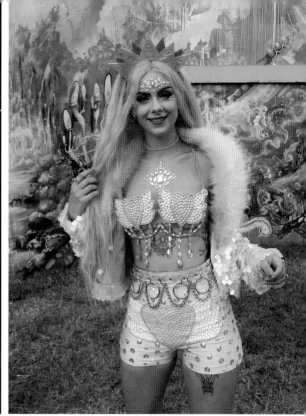
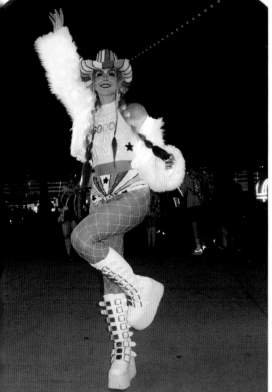
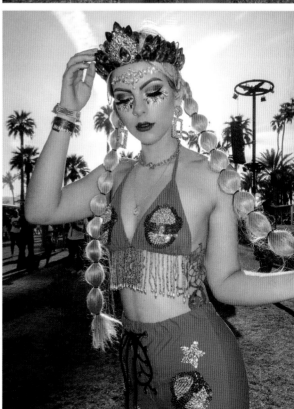

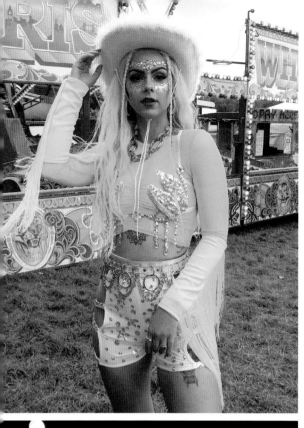
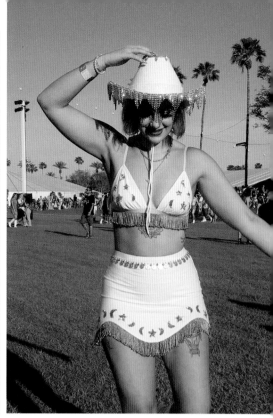
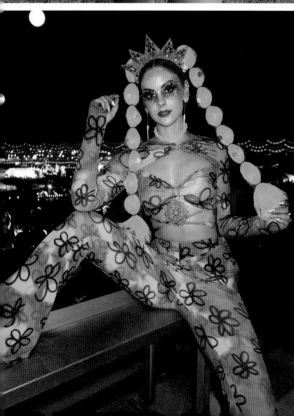
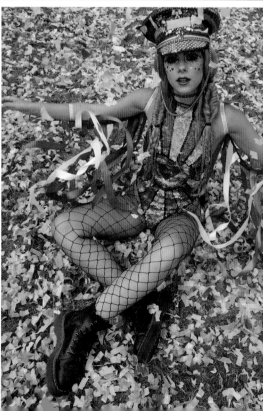

HALLOWEEN

Finally, probably my second-favourite occasion is Halloween. I feel like you'd be able to guess why… I've always been obsessed with fancy dress! Getting creative and styling themed looks and even DIY'ing pieces for the finishing touches brings me so much enjoyment. Over the years, I swear Halloween looks are becoming more imaginative, with people thinking outside of the norm. There are so many places you can take inspiration from for your costumes:

TV shows or movies	Animals	Books
Characters	Celebrities	Objects
Jobs	Food	Eras

Or you can stick to the most popular Halloween looks – typically a skeleton, witch, devil, clown, zombie, or Disney character. It depends how much money and time you want to spend on your costume. If you want something quick and easy, there are many looks you can create using clothing already in your wardrobe.

- **Goth** – wear all-black everything, statement chain, stud jewellery, fishnet tights and heavy eyeliner.

- **Sandy from Grease** – Black off-the-shoulder top, black high-waist trouser, black leather jacket, red lipstick and curly hair.

- **Euphoria** – sparkly dress and rhinestone makeup.

- **Barbie** – an iconic Barbie pink dress, heels and lipstick.

- **Devil** – all-red everything, the only purchase you might need to make is some devil horns.

- **Clueless** – a check skirt and matching blazer, knee high socks, white shirt and heels.

- **Skeleton** – this is all about the makeup, so you can pair it with an all-black outfit or paint a skeleton frame onto a white t-shirt.

- **Ariana Grande** – high ponytail, sharp eyeliner and a short puffy skater dress.

- **The Addams Family** – you've most probably got outfits to create Morticia, Wednesday, Pugsley and Gomez Addams. Why not team up with your friends on a group costume?

- **Cat** – all-black everything. Could be a black bodysuit paired with black tights. You could even make DIY cat ears from pipe cleaners.

- **Carrie** – from the Prom scene. All you need is a white dress, tons of fake blood and a tiara.

- **Ghost** – if you're happy to sacrifice a bed sheet, cut two holes and you're set!

- **A from Pretty Little Liars** – super-simple, all you need is black leggings and a hoodie.

- **Pumpkin** – classic Halloween look, it's mainly about the makeup, but you could either theme the outfit all orange or all black.

- **Witch** – another iconic Halloween costume, pull out your little black dress for this one and all you'll need to finish the look is a witch's hat, which you could make out of card.

- **Powerpuff Girls** – a cute trio costume, one of you dresses in baby blue, one pink and another green. You can even do your makeup to match.

- **A mummy** – time to raid your first aid kit in the cupboard and find those bandages. Wear a neutral outfit and wrap bandages around your whole body, securing carefully with safety pins.

- **Zombie** – grab a white shirt you don't mind donating it to the fancy dress box, tear it, cut rips and wipe some mud over it from your garden or local park. You can add ketchup on the shirt to make it look like blood, add some ripped tights or leggings, then finish with zombie makeup.

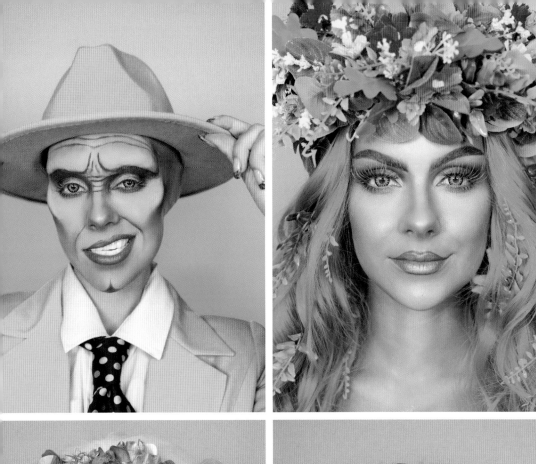
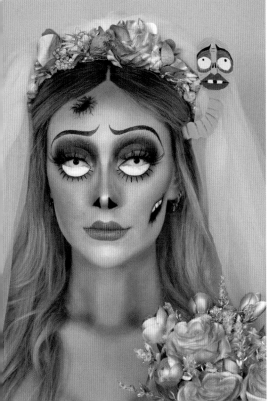
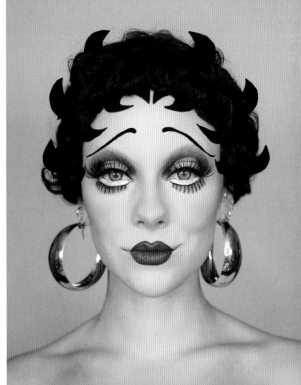

- **Pyjamas** – when else can you use the excuse to leave the house in your pyjamas and dressing gown? At least you won't have to change at the end of the night.

- **Sims** – pop on a normal outfit and DIY a green Sim symbol out of card and a headband.

These are just a handful of quick and easy last-minute ideas you can throw together with items you already have, which is great if you're wanting to be sustainable, as most often you'll only wear a Halloween costume once and pick something else the following year. If you do have more time and a budget, though, you can get super-creative with a costume. Here is some inspiration from past Halloween looks I've created.

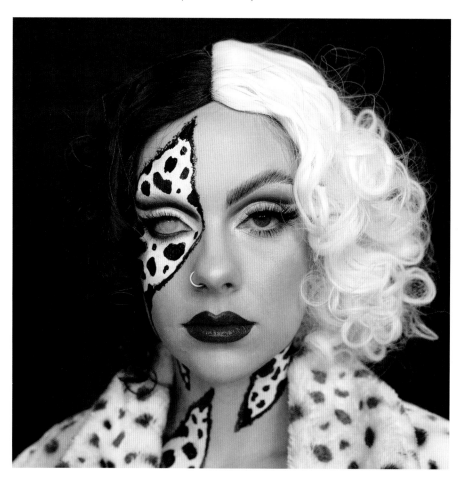

My Favourite Places to Shop

From sustainable to on trend, independent and handmade, here are my favourite places to shop:

Aurora Moon Headwear
A small, independent brand stocking handmade magical headwear from crowns to headbands, perfect for festivals and parties.

B The Label
Founded by Brooke Andrews, B The Label stocks luxury handmade clothing from dresses to co-ord sets. Think glam evening wear for nights out and holidays.

Cinta The Label
Cinta takes inspiration from adventure, vintage heirlooms, a love for whimsical but practical collections, people and spiritual journeys. They aim to bring fun, timeless pieces to your wardrobe, celebrating women of all ages! They only sell small runs and seasonal drops and have a no-waste policy.

Damson Madder
Clothing brand for men and women using organic cotton, recycled and repurposed fabrics. Ethically sourced and transparent with sustainability. From festival and holiday to wedding wear.

Easy Tiger
Easy Tiger is an independent brand about setting the trends in fashion and empowering people all over the globe while keeping it sustainable and ethical. From festival ranges to summer and autumn, their clothing is fun, bold and bright. Eco-conscious – five trees are planted for every order.

Elsie and Fred
An independent black-owned brand, founded by three siblings from Coventry, England. Their aim is to make their customers feel fierce and fun. Colourful, bold prints and eccentric clothing. They empower their community by speaking up about various

topics. They're pro-black, pro-gay, pro-liberal, pro-human. They're open about how they manufacture their clothing and are always working to be more sustainable.

Faithfull the Brand
Founded in Indonesia in 2012, Faithfull the Brand has care, quality and authenticity woven into its fabric. The brand collaborates with Bali's best manufacturers to create their handmade garments, and live and work closely with their local community. At the heart of the brand are thoughtfully produced designs that evoke a sense of summer and a spirit of travel. Faithfull is known and loved for its vintage-inspired prints, flattering shapes and unique pieces, made for sun-seekers and romantic dreamers.

Another Girl
A unique reimagining of nostalgic romance and contemporary influences. Another Girl is youthful, feminine, effortless and informed. Their signature prints and premium-quality fabrics elevate their collections and ensure longevity beyond a season. Another Girl is concerned about the planet, working with ethical factories and using recycled fabrics when possible.

Hat & Spicy
A small, independent brand upcycling party hats. Custom, bespoke, handmade to order and cruelty free.

Her Pony the Label
A brand whose core values stem from the love for what they do and kindness to everything in the process – for their makers, for their customers and for the planet. Stocking a range of ethical and limited-edition, vintage-inspired festival clothing.

Hosbjerg
Hosbjerg is a Danish fashion brand based in Copenhagen, founded by Camilla Hosbjerg. Camilla created the brand with the purpose of making good-quality designs in at affordable prices. Something she felt had been missing in the industry. 'It's important for us to dare to be innovative and different. Bright colours, funky prints and crooked details will always be a part of our collections.'

House of Sunny

An independent women's and menswear brand from Hackney, London. They create unique, timeless designs for easy, everyday wear; each product is carefully crafted to become the perfect addition to elevate any wardrobe that can transition through the seasons. Quality, eco-conscious, cruelty-free and vegan.

Jungle Club Clothing

A UK fashion brand based in Sheffield. Cute and quirky is their thing, selling everything from sunglasses and hats to clothing. Supports slow fashion and ships worldwide.

Kai Collective

Kai Collective is a London-based brand of attainable clothing with luxury aesthetics, founded by Fisayo Longe. As an OG fashion and travel blogger since 2012, Fisayo would go fabric shopping during her trips and share the outfits that she made with the fabric, leading to questions from her community about where she got her outfits from. This is how Kai was born. It's a clothing brand for women, by women. They craft clothes to make multidimensional women feel like the most confident version of themselves.

Magical Wonderland

Based in Sydney, Australia, Magical Wonderland is a fun and youthful contemporary women's festival fashion brand dedicated to the modern sparkle queen. Full of pastel colours, sequin details and trendy silhouettes, Magical Wonderland is all about expressing your individuality and inner creativity at your next festival, rave or special event!

Meshki

Founded by two architecture students with a love of fashion, the girls allude to their Persian heritage through their designs: 'Meshki is Farsi for black, and black for us embodies so much of what our brand is about.' (The darker the chocolate, the richer the taste, baby!) Meshki is a series of juxtapositions; mysterious yet bold, sleek yet sexy, subdued yet powerful. With on-trend statement designs that accentuate the female figure, the brand creates collections that scream luxe without the price tag or compromise to quality.

Molby The Label

Molby The Label is an independent, British, slow-fashion brand. Each garment is designed and handmade in a studio by a small team. You'll find fun, affordable garments, which can be dressed up or down for all occasions. The brand's aim is to focus on a more ethical way of working, by reducing fabric wastage and carbon emissions and creating high-quality, timeless garments that can be worn again and again. Each piece is handmade to order, which allows customers to make small changes to designs, whether it's custom sizing or changing the hem length, fabric or colour.

Never Fully Dressed

Founded by Lucy Aylen, NFD is a womenswear label with bold prints and multi-wear styles. Their clothing can be dressed up or down and is made for all bodies, shapes and ages. Eco-conscious and ethical, some of their clothing is made from recycled fabrics. They also have a pre-loved programme where if you want to get rid of a worn NFD item you can give it back to the brand in return for loyalty points that you can spend on their newer collections; they then sell the old garments on Depop.

Neon Rose

Home to a small independent team of women bringing you the latest trend-led pieces, designed in Manchester, UK. They celebrate femininity with a splash of fun. Think oversized collars, layered knitwear, retro prints and co-ords.

New Girl Order

Launched in 2018, NGO is your one-stop destination for all things bold, stand-out and cute. They embrace individuality and creativity, from trend-led pieces to graphic tees and bold prints.

Poster Girl

Founded by Francesca Capper and Natasha Somerville in 2017. A label manifesting confidence, ultra-femininity and referencing a direct nostalgia to the designers' upbringings. By pushing and developing surface textures, the high-gloss aesthetic of this brand is backed with sophisticated, luxurious construction techniques and quality. The brand celebrates inner confidence and femininity, making its rise within the fashion and pop-culture scene nothing short of explosive.

Shop Fluffy

An independent brand stocking handmade crochet clothing in a bright colour palette. It's fun, cute and playful. From matching sets to cardigans, this crochet clothing is made to last.

Somewhere Nowhere

An independent brand selling clothing for anyone who dares to express themselves and is fearless with colours and texture. Founded by creative duo Rex Lo and Elly Cheng. Custom-made and worldwide shipping.

Subtropic

Your one-stop shop for swimwear and festival fashion, their clothing is colourful, bold and bright. Everything is created in-house in London and is handmade to order, with a mission to do their part in creating ethical and sustainable products.

Wear To Be Seen

A small, independent brand making swimwear and clothing to order. Based in Glasgow, all designs are created in-house by designer and founder Danielle Meighan and her small team. Clothing is inspired by vintage fashion, bold prints and colour and all fabric prints are made completely exclusively, so you won't find them elsewhere. Offer customisation with changing fabrics and styles so you can find a design that suits you.

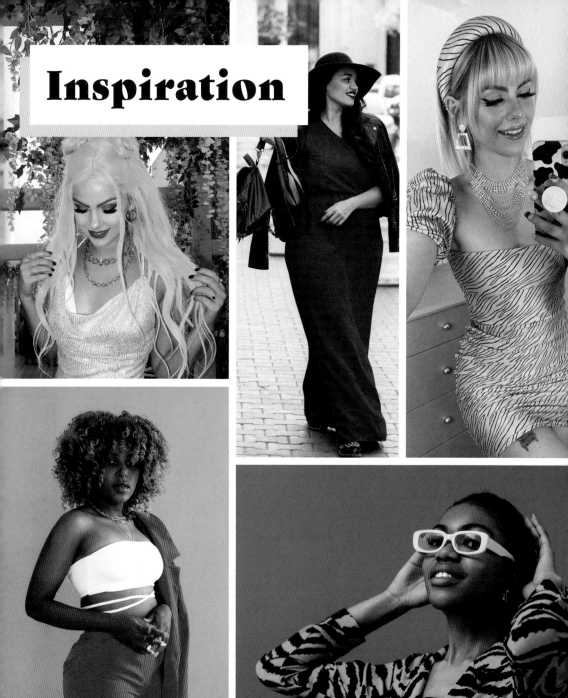

Inspiration

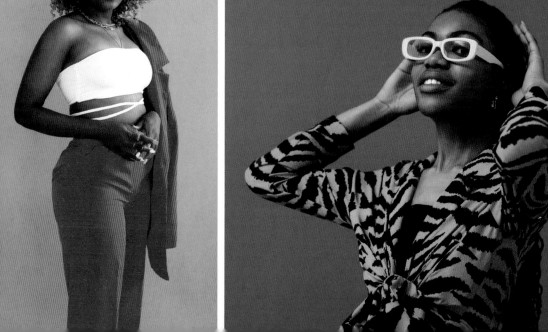

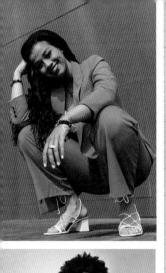
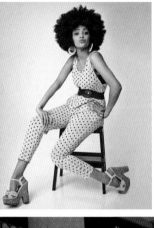
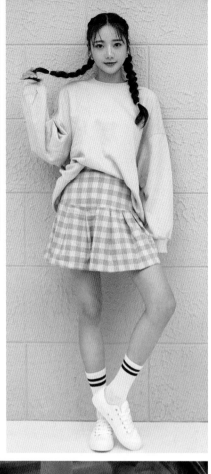
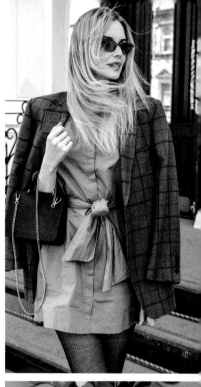
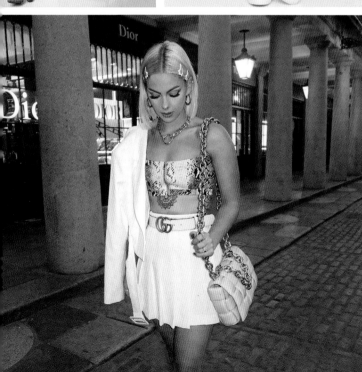
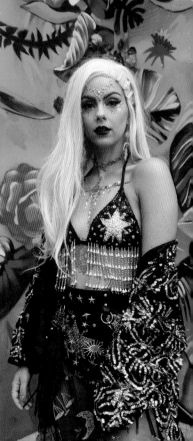

The Beauty Brands

BRAND	BEAUTY	ABOUT	COST	ONLINE/ STORE
Alkemilla	Cosmetics	Organic eco-cosmetics brand from Italy	Mid	Online
Anastasia Beverly Hills	Cosmetics	American cosmetics brand best known for their eyebrow products	High	Online, Boots
BaByliss	Hair	High-quality and stylish hair-styling tools	Mid	Online, Argos, Boots
Barry M Cosmetics	Cosmetics	On-trend, high-quality, affordable cosmetics	Affordable	Boots, Superdrug
Beauty Works	Hair	Leaders in luxury hair extensions; also offer haircare and styling tools	Mid	Online and hair salons
Beautyblender	Cosmetics	The original beauty blender makeup applicator	Mid	Online, Boots
Benefit	Cosmetics	Feel-good makeup brand, founded in San Francisco	Mid	Online, Boots own stores
Briogeo	Hair	Offers clean, natural and effective haircare products for all hair types and textures	High	Online, SpaceNK
Bumble and Bumble	Hair	Cruelty-free haircare products created by stylists working on backstage shows and shoots	High	Online, Boots, John Lewis
CeraVe	Skincare	Complete line of skincare developed with dermatologists	Affordable	Online, Boots, Superdrug
Cetaphil	Skincare	Skincare recommended by dermatologists targeted at sensitive skin	Affordable	Online, Boots, Superdrug

BRAND	BEAUTY	ABOUT	COST	ONLINE/ STORE
Charlotte Tilbury	Cosmetics	Founded by British MUA Charlotte herself. Award-winning makeup and skincare	High	Online, John Lewis, Fenwick
Chopstick Styler	Hair	Rectangular-shaped curling wand range	Mid	Online, Argos
Cinema Secrets	Cosmetics	Professional cosmetics for MUAs and makeup enthusiasts most known for their brush-cleaning range	High	Online
Claire's	Hair	Fun, on-trend hair accessories	Affordable	In store and online
Clinique	Skincare	Most known for their skincare but also offer cosmetics, toiletries and fragrances	High	Online, Boots John Lewis
Coco & Eve	Hair	Award-winning haircare, bodycare, self-tanning and skincare	High	Online, Selfridges
Coco Cosmetics by Chloe	Makeup	Makeup brand founded by an MUA and most known for their marshmallow sponge makeup applicator	Affordable	Online
Code8	Cosmetics	London-based luxury, high-performance makeup	High	Online, in store, Fenwick
Collection	Cosmetics	High-quality, easy to use, affordable makeup for every look	Affordable	Online, Boots
Coloured Raine	Cosmetics	Cruelty-free and vegan cosmetics brand with high pigmentation	Mid	Online
Crazy Lenses	Cosmetics	High-quality, affordable, contact lenses for Halloween and creative looks	Affordable	Online

BRAND	BEAUTY	ABOUT	COST	ONLINE/ STORE
Davines	Hair	Sustainable haircare brand founded in Italy and made with ingredients of natural origin	High	Online, Liberty London, in hair salons
Dermalogica	Skincare	No.1 professional skincare brand in the UK and Ireland	High	Online, John Lewis, Fenwick
Dior	Cosmetics	Designer beauty brand	High	Online, John Lewis
Dose of Colors	Cosmetics	Cruelty-free makeup brand inspired by colour and comfort; offers high-quality products with high pigment	Mid	Online
Dyson	Hair	Pioneering technology now offering haircare	High	Online, John Lewis, Currys
e.l.f. Cosmetics	Cosmetics	Affordable makeup and beauty products that are cruelty-free	Affordable	Online, Boots
ECO Style	Cosmetics	Known for their hair gel that promotes hair growth and enhances hair health	Affordable	Online
EcoTools	Cosmetics	100% cruelty-free and vegan synthetic makeup brushes, sponges, applicators and bath accessories that are both stylish and eco-friendly	Mid	Online, Boots, Superdrug
Ecooking	Cosmetics	Everyday luxury for your skin. Developed with a strong focus on the ingredients and the effect they have. Offering skincare as well as cosmetics	High	Online

BRAND	BEAUTY	ABOUT	COST	ONLINE/STORE
Elemis	Skincare	No. 1 British anti-ageing skincare with over 30 years of expertise	High	Online, John Lewis, Boots
Ere Perez	Cosmetics	Ere Perez is natural skincare and makeup made from powerful botanical ingredients for clean, conscious living	High	Online
Estée Lauder	Makeup	High-performance skincare, makeup and fragrance	High	Online, Selfridges, John Lewis
EVO Hair	Hair	Cruelty-free professional haircare and body products	Mid	Online, Boots, Superdrug
Eylure	Cosmetics	The home of false eyelashes. Eylure was created by MUAs with a passion for innovation	Affordable	Online, Boots
Faace	Skincare	Fuss-free, fast-acting skincare for all faces. From masks to treatments	Mid	Online
Face Halo	Cosmetics	Award-winning reusable makeup remover pad	Mid	Online, Boots
Faith in Nature	Hair	Award-winning natural beauty products including hair, body, skin, baby and home-care products. Ethical and cruelty-free alternatives	Affordable	Online, Boots, Holland & Barrett
Fudge Professional	Hair	From hair styling to shampoos, conditioners and treatments. Diverse products that push the boundaries	Mid	Online, Boots

BRAND	BEAUTY	ABOUT	COST	ONLINE/STORE
Garnier	Hair/skincare	Most known for haircare, skincare, sun protection and body care	Affordable	Online, Boots, Superdrug
Gen See	Cosmetics	Committed to clean, vegan and sustainable makeup	Mid	Online
ghd	Hair	Most known for their heated styling tools, from straighteners to curlers and hairdryers	High	Online, John Lewis, Selfridges
got2b	Hair	From volume and shine to hold and spikes, got2b offers the right styling products for your look	Affordable	Online, Boots, supermarkets
Hello Sunday	Skincare	Sun care meets skincare. Multi-functional SPF brand that's got you covered, come rain or shine	Mid	Online, SpaceNK
Hourglass	Cosmetics	Hourglass, the cruelty-free beauty brand, is known for its innovation and commitment to reinventing luxury cosmetics	High	Online, John Lewis, Selfridges, Harvey Nicols
Huda Beauty	Cosmetics	The store for all things makeup, skincare, fragrance, beauty tools, tips and trends founded by makeup mogul Huda Kattan	Mid-high	Online, Boots, Selfridges
INIKA	Cosmetics	INIKA has developed the world's first 100% natural skincare range infused with 5% botanical actives	Mid-high	Online
Invisibobble	Hair	invisibobble® ORIGINAL, the traceless hair ring	Affordable	Online, Boots, supermarkets

BRAND	BEAUTY	ABOUT	COST	ONLINE/STORE
KASH Beauty	Cosmetics	Makeup and beauty brand founded by well-known Irish MUA and influencer Keilidh Cashell	Mid	Online
K18	Hair	K18Peptide™ is the patented molecular breakthrough clinically proven to reverse hair damage from: bleach + color, chemical services, and heat	High	Online
Kiehl's	Skincare	Dermatologist since 1851, recommended skincare, body care, haircare, beauty products made using a variety of natural and well-sourced ingredients	High	Online, own stores, Boots, SpaceNK
KIKO Milano	Cosmetics	Established and founded in 1997 by Percassi, this Italian professional cosmetics brand features a range of cutting-edge makeup, face and body products	Affordable–mid	Online, own stores
KISS	Cosmetics	Offers the look of lash extensions in minutes with their false eyelashes	Affordable	Online, Boots, Superdrug
L'Oréal	Cosmetics	The world's largest cosmetics company offers makeup, skincare and hair products	Affordable	Online, Boots, Superdrug
La Roche-Posay	Skincare	Range of skincare products, backed by science, specifically formulated to maximise the health and beauty of your skin	Mid	Online, Boots, Superdrug
Lancôme	Cosmetics	Luxurious makeup, skincare and fragrance	High	Online, John Lewis

BRAND	BEAUTY	ABOUT	COST	ONLINE/STORE
Lily Lolo	Cosmetics	Clean cosmetics brand offering makeup and brushes. Gentle to skin and bismuth-free	Affordable-mid	Online
Lime Crime	Cosmetics	Vegan and cruelty-free makeup and hair brand that aims to inspire and express	Mid	Online
Living Proof	Hair	Hair products that are cruelty-free, paraben-free and silicone-free, for visibly healthier hair	High	Online, SpaceNK
MAC Cosmetics	Cosmetics	Most known for their Studio Fix range. A beauty and makeup brand made by artists	Mid–high	Online, own stores, John Lewis, Selfridges
Made By Mitchell	Cosmetics	Made by Mitchell offers a fresh, new take on cruelty-free cosmetics, packing more pigment, quality and serious value for money	Mid	Online
Makeup Revolution	Cosmetics	Award-winning makeup, skincare and haircare. High-quality, cruelty-free and affordable	Affordable	Online, Boots, Superdrug
Mane 'n Tail	Hair	Haircare originally formulated for horses and discovered by humans	Affordable	Online, Boots
Maybelline	Cosmetics	Most known for their affordable cosmetics, skincare and fragrances	Affordable	Online, Boots, Superdrug
Milk Makeup	Cosmetics	Clean, cruelty-free, vegan makeup. Striving to make the best milk beauty products with good ingredients	Mid	Online, Selfridges

BRAND	BEAUTY	ABOUT	COST	ONLINE/STORE
Morphe	Cosmetics	Morphe was born in 2008 among the artists and influencers in Los Angeles. Most known for their eye palettes	Mid	Online, own stores
MUA Makeup Academy	Cosmetics	Your go-to brand for high-quality, affordable makeup, cosmetics and beauty products. All products are 100% vegan and cruelty-free	Affordable	Online, Superdrug
Mykitco.	Cosmetics	Professional makeup brushes and accessories designed by makeup artist James Molloy for makeup artists and makeup lovers	High	Online
NATorigin	Cosmetics	Allergy UK-approved, the NATorigin range is designed with sensitive skin and eyes in mind, as well as using natural and organic ingredients	Mid	Online
Nicmac Beauty	Cosmetics	Nicmac Beauty is a UK-based and -formulated makeup brand. 100% Vegan and animal cruelty-free while creating new ways of being sustainable	Mid	Online
NIOXIN Professional	Hair	NIOXIN's highly effective ranges strengthen, nourish and repair thinning hair from the scalp, which is the foundation for healthy, thicker, fuller hair	Mid	Online, Boots

BRAND	BEAUTY	ABOUT	COST	ONLINE/ STORE
NYX Professional Makeup	Cosmetics	American makeup brand from LA that promotes self-expression. Affordable, highly pigmented and long-lasting	Affordable	Online, Superdrug
OFRA Cosmetics	Cosmetics	Iinternationally recognised in the beauty industry, specialising in highlighter and liquid lipstick	Mid	Online
OGX	Hair	Affordable salon-inspired haircare for all hair types and textures	Affordable	Online, supermarkets, Superdrug
OLAPLEX	Hair	Haircare using patented OLAPLEX® Bond Building Technology working on a molecular level to repair damaged and broken bonds	High	Online, SpaceNK
Ole Henriksen	Skincare	Skincare that promotes radiant, glowing skin	High	Online, Boots
OSMO	Hair	OSMO® is a leading collection of professional colour, care and styling products designed to give stylists and barbers the power and confidence to create	Mid	Online, Sally Beauty
OUAI	Hair	OUAI haircare by celebrity hairstylist Jen Atkin. Award-winning hair, body and lifestyle products	Mid–high	Online, SpaceNK, Selfridges
PerfectlaceWig	Hair	Specialises in all kinds of high-quality human hair wigs with worldwide shipping	High	Online

BRAND	BEAUTY	ABOUT	COST	ONLINE/STORE
Real Techniques	Cosmetics	Produces professional-quality makeup brushes, makeup sponges, applicators and accessories that are both stylish and functional	Mid	Online, Boots
Red Carpet FX	Cosmetics	Professional makeup, face and body paints, special FX supplies, prosthetics and brushes	Mid–high	Online
Redken	Hair	Offering professional haircare, hairstyling and colour	Mid–high	Online, Sally Beauty
Revamp	Hair	Salon-quality heated styling tools featuring Progloss Oils technology	Mid–high	Online
Revlon Professional	Hair	The home for professional hair colouring, cutting and products	Mid	Online
Rimmel London	Cosmetics	UK's no. 1 makeup brand promoting individuality and self-expression	Affordable	Online, Superdrug
ROEN Beauty	Cosmetics	They promise to bring you clean beauty products that are high performing, luxe and easy to use. Cruelty free, vegan and gluten free	High	Online
Schwarzkopf	Hair	A hair cosmetics brand offering haircare, colour and styling products for over 120 years	Affordable	Online, Boots, Supermarkets
Shiseido	Cosmetics	Japanese beauty brand offering high performance skincare, luxe makeup and fragrance	High	Online, Boots

BRAND	BEAUTY	ABOUT	COST	ONLINE/ STORE
SILKE London	Hair	Founder Maria took inspiration from her Caribbean heritage of traditional hair wrapping and created SILKE London. Offering 100% silk haircare products as she found that wrapping her hair in 100% silk had incredible results	High	Online
Sleek MakeUP	Cosmetics	Offering highly pigmented and affordable cosmetics from eye palettes to highlighters and lipstick	Affordable	Online, Boots
Smashbox Cosmetics	Cosmetics	LA cosmetics brand known for their iconic The Original Photo Finish primer	Mid	Online
Sophie Hannah Hair	Hair	Haircare and hair colour brand founded by Sophie Hannah. Cruelty-free, vegan and sustainable	Mid	Online
Spectrum Collections	Cosmetics	Makeup that is gluten-free, cruelty-free, vegan. Suitable for all ages, skin tones and occasions. Made for both day and night	High	Online, House of Fraser
Sunday Riley	Skincare	Skincare that is powered by science and balanced by botanicals, for total skin improvement and wellness	High	Online, Space NK
Tangle Teezer	Hair	Tangle Teezer are the famous detangling hairbrush brand	Affordable	Online, John Lewis, Superdrug

BRAND	BEAUTY	ABOUT	COST	ONLINE/ STORE
Tatti Lashes	Cosmetics	Tatti Lashes specialise in the highest-quality, handmade luxury lashes ranging from strip lashes to professional lash tech trays	Affordable– mid	Online
The INKEY List	Hair/ skincare	Knowledge-powered skincare and hair products	Affordable	Online
The Quick Flick	Cosmetics	Beauty innovations for everyday people, most known for their winged eyeliner stamp. Cruelty-free, vegan and non-toxic	Mid	Online, Superdrug
TIGI Bed Head	Hair	Bed Head is an innovative range of haircare and styling products, created by hairdressers to deliver endless creative possibilities	Mid	Online, Superdrug
Too Faced	Cosmetics	Innovative cruelty-free makeup and skincare offering trendsetting products	Mid–high	Online, John Lewis, Selfridges
Ultra Violette	Skincare	Founded in Australia, Ultra Violette is redefining sunscreen with SPF	High	Online
Urban Decay	Cosmetics	Badass cruelty-free, high-pigment makeup. Colour that goes all day and lasts all night	High	Online, Boots
VIEVE	Cosmetics	High-performance, purposeful and universal makeup, founded by makeup artist, Jamie Genevieve	High	Online
VO5	Hair	Hair styling products that meet your everyday needs	Affordable	Online, Savers, Superdrug, supermarkets

BRAND	BEAUTY	ABOUT	COST	ONLINE/STORE
Wet n Wild	Cosmetics	Based in Los Angeles, Wet n Wild launched in 1979 and continue to deliver quality products at affordable prices	Affordable	Online, Boots
Wet Brush	Hair	Pain-free brushing for every occasion and hair type	Mid	Online, Boots
Wishful Skin	Skincare	Gentle, simple, cruelty-free skincare born from influencer Huda Kattan, who struggles with her own skin	Mid–high	Online
ZAO	Cosmetics	For a beauty that takes care of your skin and nature, ZAO has created for you 100% natural cosmetics, organic* and vegan certified	Mid	Online
ZOEVA	Cosmetics	ZOEVA is dedicated to celebrating individual beauty, providing you with high-quality makeup and tools	Mid	Online

Acknowledgements

To all the individuals who follow me across social media, this book would not have been possible without you. You've watched me create beauty and fashion content for the best part of a decade, supported me, allowed me to be true to myself and grow as a person. This book is for you; and I hope you find it inspiring and enjoy reading it as much as I enjoyed writing it.

To my biggest supporter, my husband Robin. You have been on this journey from the beginning, from helping me with shooting outfits for my blog on your days off, to now coming on board full time. We make a great team and I love having you by my side on this journey. You support every decision I make and when my mental health has been a struggle, you've got me through. I appreciate those dog walks with you after hours spent writing! You're an amazing listener and I'm grateful for those times you offer a different perspective and opinion.

To my fur babies Luna and Shadow, I couldn't leave you two out. You kept me company through all the book-writing days and for that I am truly grateful.

To my late Dad, thank you for passing on your passion and drive. You may no longer be with us, but you inspire me in everything that I do. You were a hardworking and dedicated man, and your love for photography encouraged me to pursue a degree in Fashion with Photography, which then developed into becoming a full-time content creator. I'm sad that I can't share this book with you, but I know how proud you'd be of me.

To my Mum, we've had our fair share of up and downs but I'm thankful for how you have always allowed me to be myself. You never judged the way I dressed growing up or my ever-changing hair colour. You supported me with every decision I made in regard to choosing what to study and then picking a career path. You enabled my creativity to flourish.

To Katie, having you as a sister, who is also an amazing, trained MUA, has helped me tremendously. Our chats, from makeup brushes to brows, has offered me insightful tips and tricks to practise, learn and develop. You're another big supporter of mine; I'm lucky to be able to call you my best friend and grateful to always have you on the end of the phone.

To HarperCollins and in particular Lydia, thank you for believing in me and bringing me on board to write this book. You have given me such an amazing opportunity and seamless experience. You have brought my passion, voice and creativity to life and you're sharing it for all to see and be inspired by.

Thorsons
An imprint of HarperCollins*Publishers*
1 London Bridge Street
London SE1 9GF

www.harpercollins.co.uk

HarperCollins*Publishers*
Macken House, 39/40 Mayor Street Upper
Dublin 1, D01 C9W8, Ireland

First published by HarperCollins*Publishers* 2023

1 3 5 7 9 10 8 6 4 2

A catalogue record of this book is available from the British Library

ISBN 978-0-00-855519-1

Printed and bound at PNB, Latvia

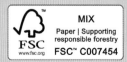